Yoga to Stay Young

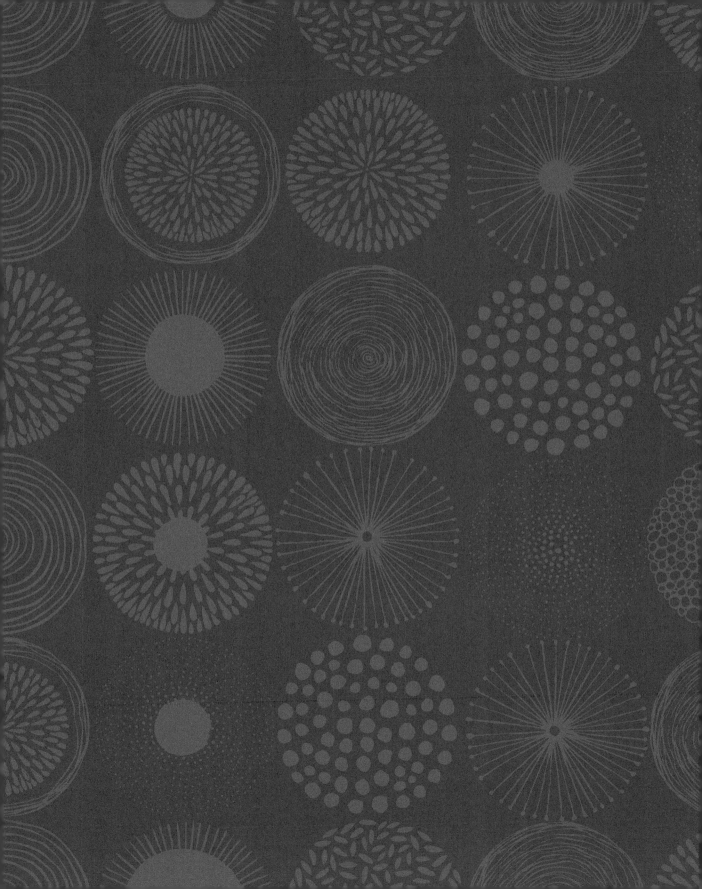

YOGA
TO STAY
YOUNG

SIMPLE POSES TO KEEP YOU
FLEXIBLE, STRONG, and PAIN-FREE

RACHEL SCOTT

ROCKRIDGE
PRESS

Interior and Cover Designer: Tricia Jang
Art Producer: Sara Feinstein
Editor: Andrea Leptinsky
Production Editor: Matt Burnett
Illustrations © 2019 Christy Ni, cover, p. 30-34, 38-42, 44, 46, 48, 50-52, 54-55, 58-60, 64-65, 67-73, 75-78, 82-85, 88-90, 92-93, 100-119, 122-128, 130-143, 146-160, 162-165, 168, 170-186, 188-189. All other illustrations used under license from Shutterstock.com.
Author Photo: © Kevin Clark

ISBN: Print 978-1-64152-453-7 | Ebook 978-1-64152-454-4

R0

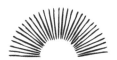

This book is dedicated to
my mom and dad, Cheryl and Bill.
I love you both very much.

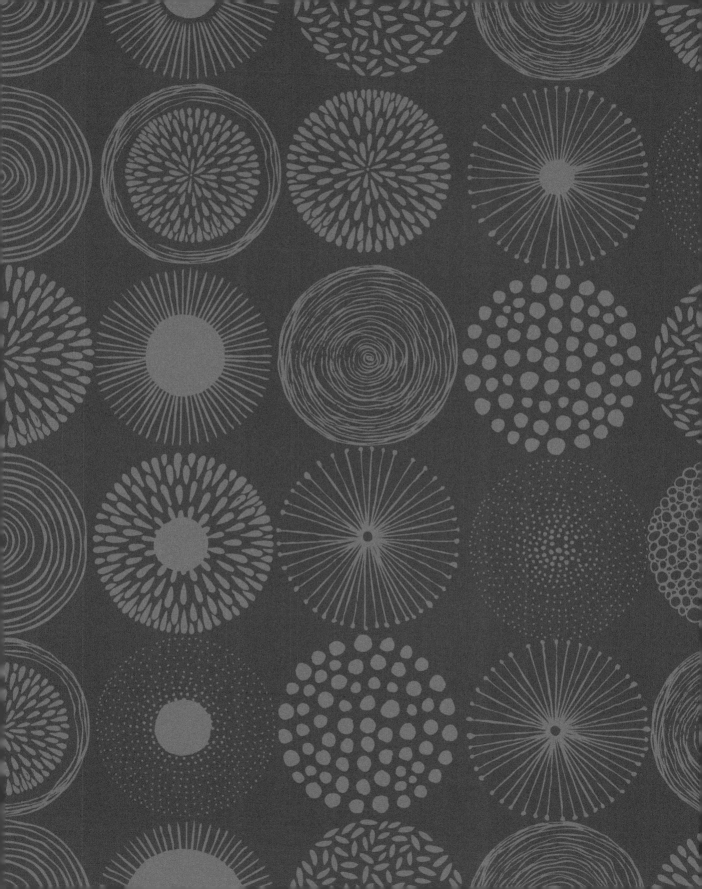

CONTENTS

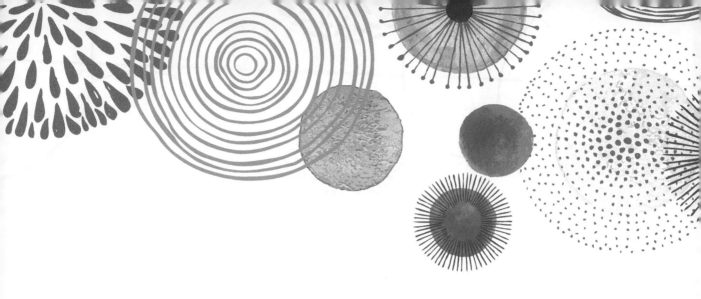

INTRODUCTION

I STARTED YOGA IN 1998 while I was living in New York City and struggling to become a working actor. Watching as my anxiety and stress levels increased, a friend offered some advice: "Try yoga. Just see what you think." I took my first class in a small studio just off Union Square. Back in those days, yoga seemed shrouded in mystery. Would there be incense burning? Would I have to chant? Would I be doing strange breathing exercises or have to tie myself into a pretzel?

To my surprise, the class was welcoming and accessible, and I didn't have to do any contortions! After my first class, I left the studio feeling grounded, connected to myself, and less anxious than I'd been in months. At that moment, I realized that yoga could be a valuable resource for supporting my mental and physical health.

When I went to graduate school in San Francisco, yoga helped me feel steady through late nights, crazy rehearsal schedules, and the challenges of earning my MFA. After completing my studies, I returned to New York City and rejoined my home yoga studio. When I found out that one of my good friends was earning her yoga teaching certification, I was consumed with jealousy (which was, admittedly, not very yogic of me). Recognizing my deep desire to learn more about the practice and its philosophy, I signed up for my first yoga teacher training.

Within a few years, I had completed two 500-hour level yoga teacher trainings, an additional 200-hour certification, and several workshops. I'd also begun apprenticing as a teacher trainer. The rest is history! I became the director of Teachers College for

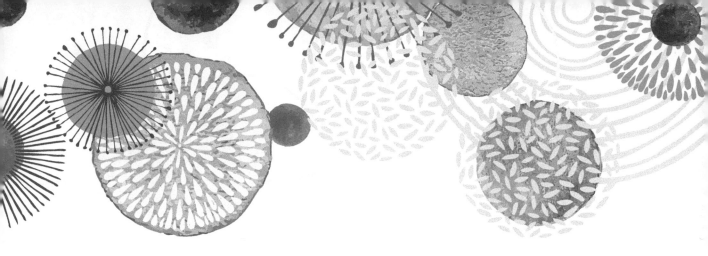

Yoga, where I helped build their teacher training department from the ground up. I have since taught more than 4,000 hours of yoga teacher training, mentored and trained hundreds of students, written three books, and launched my career as an educational consultant and coach for studios and teachers worldwide.

I firmly believe that yoga is a transformational tool that can help anyone cultivate strength, flexibility, and mindfulness. Yoga doesn't have to be "fancy" to be good. In fact, the simplest poses—done well—can deliver extraordinary results.

In this book, I will share some of my favorite poses and simple sequences. These postures can help you feel stronger and more flexible and vibrant at any age. Each pose will include variations and modifications so that you can amp up the intensity or dial it back, depending on your individual needs. Ultimately, yoga is a very personal practice; every body is different, and you are encouraged to modify the practice so it supports your body and lifestyle. Part of developing your own practice will be exploring what feels good for you rather than looking for a "one size fits all" solution.

By using this book, you can expect to increase your stamina and balance. But the benefits of yoga aren't just physical; your practice can help you sleep better, feel less stressed, cultivate mindfulness, and develop a greater sense of equanimity in your daily life.

I look forward to taking the journey with you!

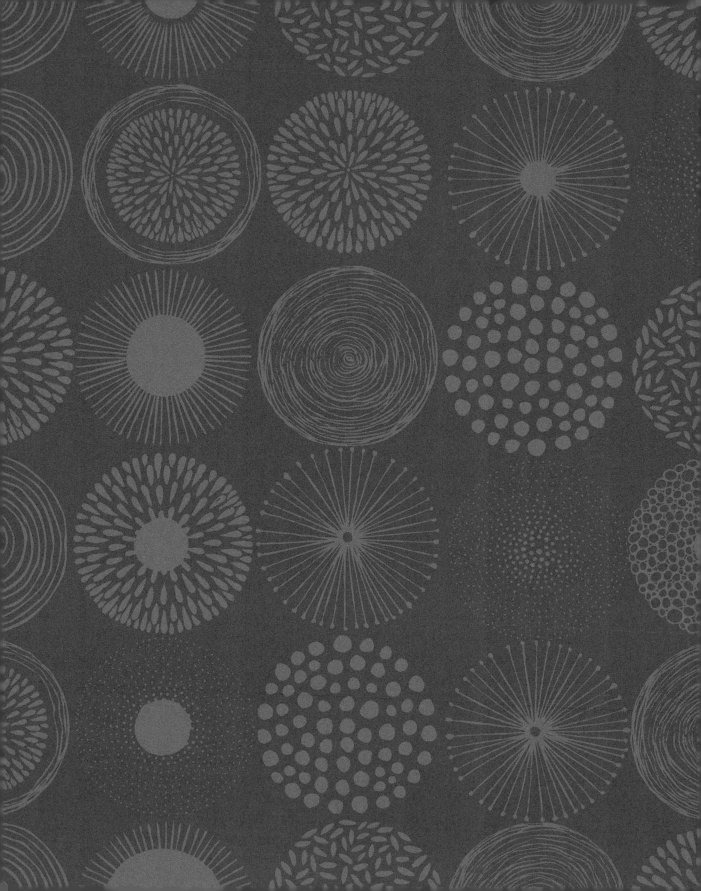

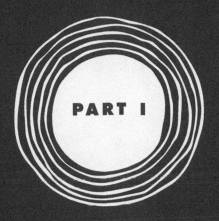

PART I

THE SCIENCE

Yoga is an ancient practice of meditation and movement that began more than 5,000 years ago in Northwest India and Pakistan. Often defined as "union," yoga is a tool for uniting the various aspects of ourselves—mental, physical, and emotional—so we can experience a greater sense of health and well-being. In North America, we tend to practice postural yoga, where we move the body into different shapes and poses. But it may surprise you to know that yoga has many different branches and styles of practice, and some of them don't involve movement at all. Regardless of the practice style, the ultimate goal of yoga is to help the practitioner calm their mind and enjoy a better sense of health and wellness.

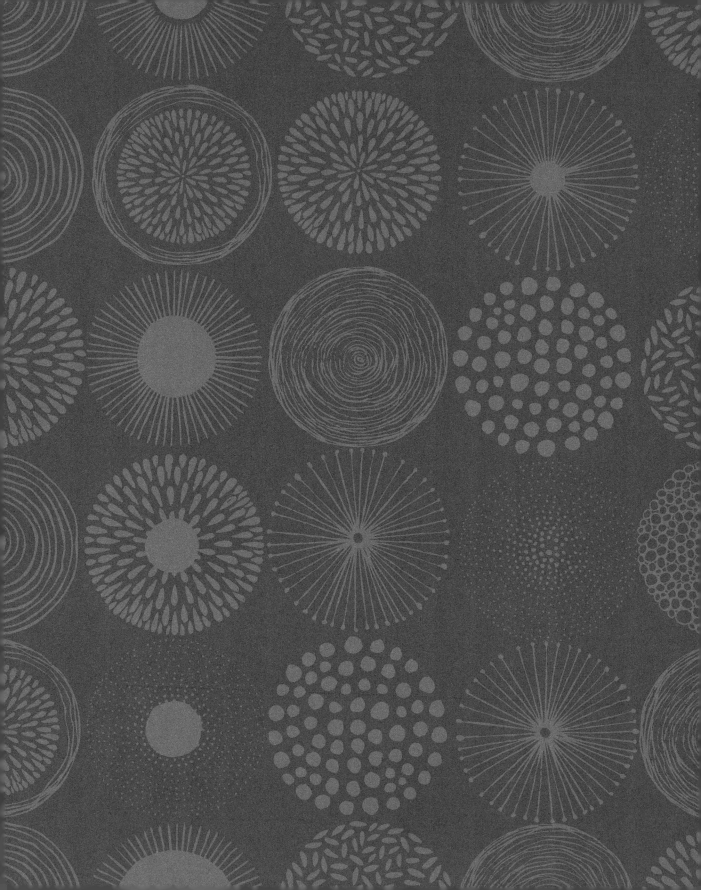

In postural yoga, we use mindful, physical movement as a tool for becoming present. Now, you may be thinking, "I was told to go to yoga class to help my low back!" and yes, it will likely do that. There are many physical benefits to postural yoga that make it popular for folks who want to improve their mobility, balance, and health issues. And added to the health and wellness package is the (not so visible) impact that yoga can have on your mind and nervous system.

Yoga gained popularity in North America during the 1960s, when spiritually curious thinkers began to travel to India in search of meaning. One particular teacher, Krishnamacharya, became very influential in the development of North American yoga. Two of his students—B. K. S. Iyengar and Pattabhi Jois—taught thousands of Westerners, who then returned to North America to spread his teachings.

Since the 1960s, yoga has gradually evolved from a fringe spiritual practice to an accessible and mainstream tool for health and mindfulness. While there are now hundreds (if not thousands) of yoga styles, most of them have evolved from the teachings of Krishnamacharya. Some popular styles include Iyengar yoga (the yoga style developed by Iyengar), Ashtanga yoga (a powerful, challenging yoga style originally developed by Jois), hot yoga, and hatha yoga. Hatha yoga is an umbrella term for many styles, but it generally refers to a slower technique that incorporates mindful alignment. In this book, we will be practicing hatha yoga.

In yoga, we move through shapes (poses) called asanas. In the original language of yoga, Sanskrit, *asana* means "seat" or "pose." It originally described the kind of meditation pose you would assume for your mindfulness practice; now, it means any shape practiced in a yoga class. A yoga sequence is simply a series of yoga poses put together in a row.

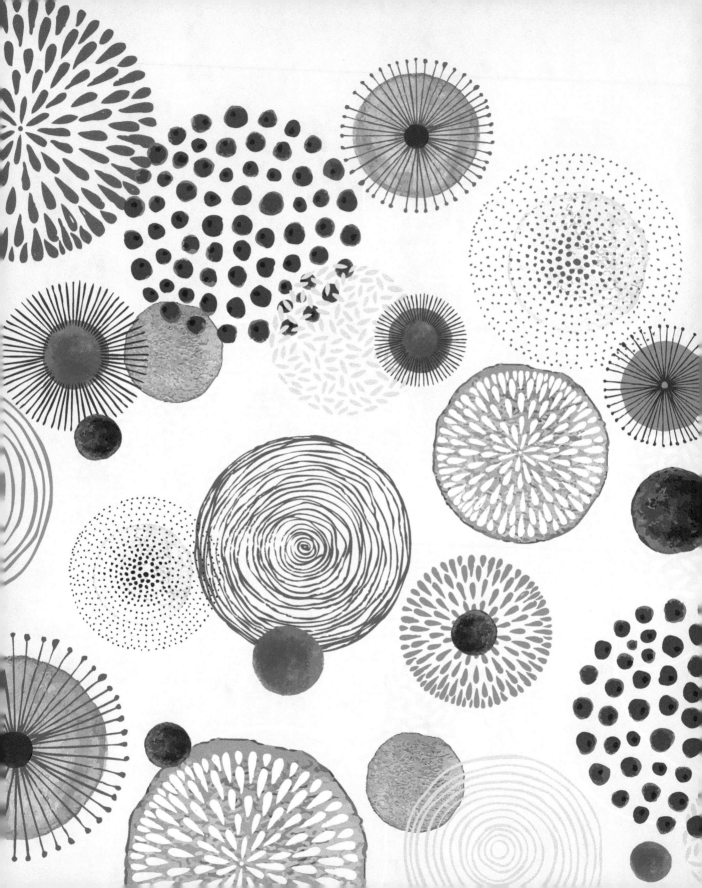

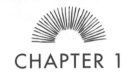

CHAPTER 1

Why Yoga Works

KNOW YOUR MUSCLES

There are four kinds of tissue in the body: nervous tissue (including the brain, spinal cord, and peripheral nervous system), epithelial tissue (for skin and linings), connective tissue (collagenous tissue that holds the body together), and muscle tissue. Muscle tissue's specialized ability to contract makes it ideal for producing force and creating movement.

TYPES OF MUSCLE TISSUE

You have three different types of muscle tissue: cardio, smooth, and skeletal. Cardio cells comprise the tissues of your heart and are designed for endurance. To appreciate just how hard your heart works, try opening and closing your fist once per second for sixty seconds. Unlike your heart, the muscles in your hand will quickly tire.

Smooth muscle is involuntary—meaning you don't consciously choose to activate it—and helps push fluids and solids internally through your body. For example, smooth muscle helps you swallow, propels food along your digestive tract, and allows your arteries to pump blood through your body.

As yoga practitioners, we are most keenly interested in the third category of muscle tissue: skeletal muscle. Skeletal muscle facilitates the movement of

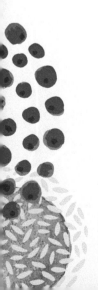

your bones at joints. Unlike cardiac and smooth muscle, most skeletal muscles are voluntary. The fibers of skeletal muscle are also usually striated so that bundles of cells can line up and work together to create force in a particular direction. Not only do your skeletal muscles allow you to walk across the room or bust out a yoga pose, they also support your posture, orient you in gravity, and regulate your sphincters (thank goodness).

STRUCTURE OF MUSCLES: BUNDLES IN BUNDLES

The tiniest component of a muscle is a small, threadlike structure called a myofibril. Thousands of myofibrils are bundled together to form a muscle fiber. These muscle fibers are then bundled together and encased in connective tissue to form fascicles. The fascicles are then bundled again (in more connective tissue) to form what we commonly think of as a "muscle." On its own, muscle tissue is surprisingly delicate. But the connective tissue provides the muscle tissue with the structural integrity necessary to do its work.

HOW YOU MOVE: JOINTS

All movement happens at joints, which are found where two bones meet. Muscles cross joints and insert into the bone via connective tissue called a tendon. The tendon is actually a continuous extension of the connective tissue that has been encasing all the bundled layers of your muscle tissue. So, when you are working your muscles, you're also working your connective tissue. When a muscle contracts, it pulls the two bones closer together and creates movement.

Let's look at an example of a muscle at work. Imagine your bicep brachii, the muscle in your upper arm that's engaged when you do a bicep curl or bend your elbow. The bicep inserts below your elbow, and then again at the top of your humerus and in your shoulder joint. When you engage this muscle and the fibers contract, they pull your lower arm toward your upper arm, which will bend your elbow (and may also cause an impressive bulge!).

HOW MUSCLES CONTRACT: THE SLIDING FILAMENT MODEL

A muscle's unique ability to contract begins at the cellular level. Myofibrils (the small units of muscles described on page 6) are composed of even smaller segments called sarcomeres, which contain two proteins: actin and myosin. When stimulated by the nervous system, these proteins use calcium and ATP (energy) to bind temporarily together, causing the sarcomere to contract. This is called the sliding filament model of muscle contraction because the filaments of actin and myosin slide against each other to shorten the sarcomere. When a whole lot of sarcomeres contract together at the same time, the muscle contracts and movement occurs.

WHY MOVEMENT IS SO DARN GOOD FOR YOU: MUSCLES AND JOINTS

Your body is designed to move.

Our modern, sedentary lifestyle is taking a toll on our health, and its negative effects are exacerbated over time. As we age, we begin to lose muscle mass (sarcopenia), which can lead to frailty and loss of functionality.

Yoga can help improve the aging process by strengthening and stretching our muscles. Consistent exercise and strength training can offset muscle loss, enabling us to maintain strength, balance, and coordination as we get older. Stretching also counteracts spinal compression, which can cause low back and joint pain. Low back pain is often caused by lumbar flexion (rounding of the low back), which is exacerbated by chronic muscular tightness in the hips. Yoga poses like Adho Mukha Svanasana (Downward Facing Dog, see page 65) actively work to lengthen the spine and create healthy traction. Yoga also includes many forward folds that stretch the hamstrings. These postures can relieve back pain by slackening the chronic tightness through the back line of the body that causes spinal compression.

Yoga can also support joint health. When stimulated by movement, the synovial joints in your body (such as your hip, knee, shoulder, elbow, and fingers) secrete synovial fluid, which lubricates your joints. Yoga is a unique physical practice because—unlike jogging or biking—it encourages your joints to work through their full range of movement in multiple directions. For example, when you ride a bike, you may only move your thigh forward and backward in the hip joint (flexion and extension), whereas a yoga sequence will also ask your thigh to externally and internally rotate, abduct, and adduct. By mobilizing your joints, yoga encourages the connective tissue around your joint (the joint capsule) to remain supple and functional.

Yoga is also a low-impact movement practice that puts less stress on the joints. For anyone with joint issues like arthritis or inflammation, high-impact movements (e.g., jogging or jumping) may exacerbate their pain. In yoga, you get all the benefits of working out your joints without the compressive impact.

WHY MOVEMENT IS SO DARN GOOD FOR YOU: CIRCULATION

In addition to supporting muscular health, movement helps your cardiovascular and lymphatic systems function at their best.

Healthy blood flow is essential to well-being. Blood is like your body's internal river, transporting cellular nutrients and waste where they need to go. When blood flow is sluggish, it's as if your internal river has become clogged. When you move, your heart rate and blood flow increase in order to supply your cells with the oxygen they need to function, which keeps your inner river flowing freely. In addition, your muscles mechanically squeeze and release your blood vessels, which supports the circulatory system to return blood to the heart.

The cells in your body float in a substance called the extracellular matrix (ECM), which is like your own internal ocean. The ECM is pulled through the lymphatic system to be cleansed of bacteria or other unsavory waste. But the lymphatic system relies on your physical movement in order to function as it should. Without movement, your internal ocean starts to look more like a stagnant pond. Movement practices like yoga help swirl your internal ocean and keep it clear and vibrant.

Studies Consistently Reveal Benefits

Yoga has long been known to have a positive impact on aging by improving postural health and physical issues like balance. But recent studies are shedding new light on how exercise supports healthy aging at the cellular level. A study published in the 2019 *Annual Review of Physiology* showed that just one exercise session can help support mitochondrial biogenesis—the growth and division of mitochondria (tiny organelles that help regulate muscle health)—which gives hope that some of the more harmful effects of aging could be slowed or even reversed through exercise (Hood, 2019).

Yoga may also have a positive impact on non-strength-related aging issues. For example, exercise may help ward off metabolic issues such as insulin resistance and diabetes (Cartee, 2016). A recent study published in *Complementary Therapies in Clinical Practice* even revealed that yoga may be an effective support for conditions such as chronic tinnitus, aka ear ringing (Niedziałek, 2019).

So, not only can yoga support the health of your muscular and circulatory systems, but it can benefit your body at the cellular level as well.

Meditation and Mindfulness

Humans have practiced meditation for thousands of years, and now, scientific research is validating the potency of mindfulness as a tool for self-regulation, health, and wellness.

Health isn't just about your muscles and bones; your nervous system is the master conductor of your body and plays an essential role in managing functions such as heart rate, blood pressure, digestion, hormones, coordination, and movement. Basically, your nervous system helps manage every aspect of your feeling, moving, and thinking.

Often, when we think of our physical health, things like physical conditioning, diet, or muscular strength come to mind. But now, we know that a wellness regime is incomplete if we aren't also taking the nervous system into consideration.

The nervous system has two subdivisions: the sympathetic and parasympathetic nervous systems. The sympathetic nervous system governs our "fight, flight, freeze, and fawn" response when we feel threatened. Once it kicks in, the sympathetic nervous system tries to protect us by increasing our heart rate and blood pressure and dumping a whole bunch of stress hormones into our bloodstream. While this survival response may have been useful when we were in danger of being eaten by tigers, these days it gets triggered by honking cars and irritating e-mails. These disturbances chronically activate our sympathetic nervous system, which can lead to harmful effects on our health over time.

In contrast, the parasympathetic nervous system has a positive effect on our overall health. It helps lower our heart rate and blood pressure and support functions like repair, digestion, memory, and maintenance. Unfortunately, we can't just manually flick on our parasympathetic nervous system like a light switch—but we do have control over our breathing, which can act like a circuit breaker and help us change gears.

Through practicing the mindful breathing techniques found in yoga, we can indirectly help move our bodies from a sympathetic to a parasympathetic state. When we slow down and regulate our breath, we induce a "relaxation response" that can slow the heart rate, reduce blood pressure, regulate hormones, and divert energy to other vital functions such as cell repair, digestion, and healing.

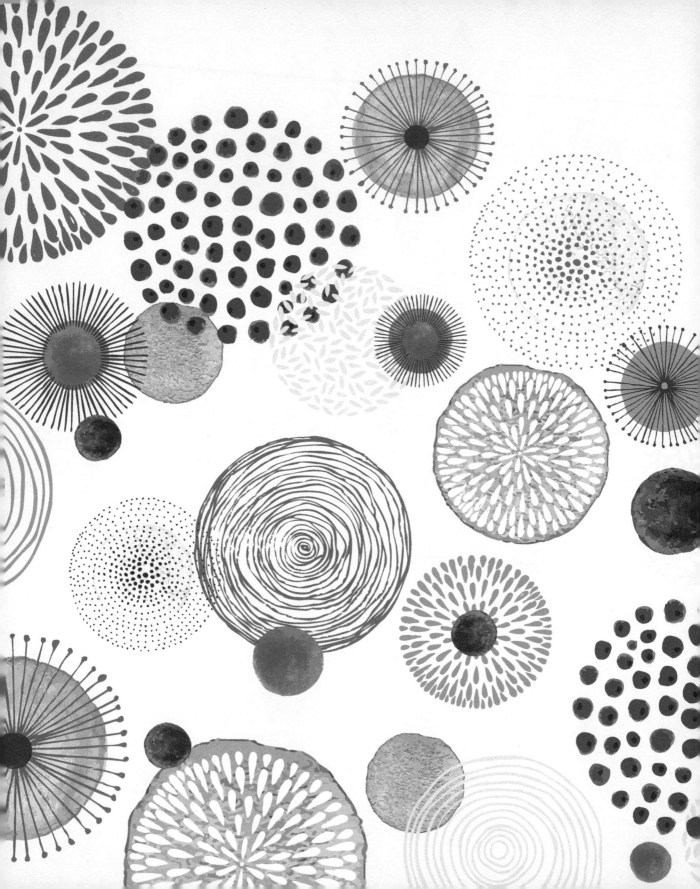

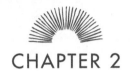

CHAPTER 2

Proper Yoga Techniques

CHOOSE A SPACE

One of the wonderful things about yoga is that you can practice it almost anywhere, anytime. When I've visited family, I've done plenty of practices right in the middle of my sister's living room. Yoga doesn't require any fancy equipment—all you need is enough room to roll out your mat. Although you will get better feedback from your hands and feet if your mat is on a firm surface like a hardwood floor, rolling your mat out on a carpet can be nice if you have sensitive joints.

While you can practice yoga almost anywhere, it can also be rewarding to set up a dedicated practice space in your home. Take a few minutes to prepare a healing environment. Clearing the clutter or putting out a nice plant or candle can make a space feel peaceful and special. Set the room to a comfortable temperature, keeping in mind that at the end of the practice you will be lying still for several minutes and may get cooler (having a cozy blanket nearby can help with this).

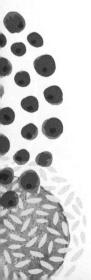

WEAR SOMETHING COMFORTABLE

You don't need to wear anything fancy for yoga. All you need are comfortable clothes that allow a full range of movement through your legs and shoulders; fitness clothes like a sweat suit or leggings work well. Yoga is usually practiced without socks for better proprioceptive feedback (body awareness) through the feet. However, if you tend to get cold, feel free to keep your socks on as long as you don't slide.

CLEAR YOUR MIND

Before beginning your practice, take a few minutes to clear your mind. Find a comfortable seated position and sit up straight with a tall spine (either on your mat or in a chair) and enjoy several deep, calming breaths. Take a few moments to set a simple intention for your practice, such as, "stay present," or "enjoy my body," or "relax." I like to invite my students to "make a transition from thinking to feeling" in order to move from the busyness of the mind into the sensations and presence of the body. Use this time to scan your body for any undue tension through your shoulders, neck, and jaw, and to relax and create space for how you are feeling.

WHAT MAKES A GOOD POSE?

While poses have a wide variety of shapes and positions, there are some commonalities that will help you do a pose properly.

A STRONG FOUNDATION. Every yoga pose starts on the ground. When you come into your posture, take special care to establish your base properly. Although this will usually be your feet, you will sometimes also use your hands. To create a stable foundation, anchor the four corners of your feet (base of the big toe, base of the pinkie toe, inner and outer heel) evenly. Rooting your feet equally will ensure that your arches are active and engaged, which assists in creating proper action through your legs. If you are rooting on your hands, make sure to root through the base of your index knuckle to avoid overcompressing your outer wrist.

STABILITY AND EASE. In yoga philosophy, asana (see page 3) has two essential ingredients: stability and ease. If we are stressed and tensed in a posture, then we are missing the ease. And if we are too relaxed and unengaged, we are missing stability. In your practice, try to cultivate both in every pose.

ALIGNMENT. When you practice, you want to keep your body aligned in a way that supports your weight to move optimally through your bones and joints. Generally, this means "stacking" your bones. For example, when standing in Tadasana (a pose where you stand upright with your feet hip distance apart and parallel), make sure that your weight is even in all four corners of both feet and that your hips are stacked over your heels so you're not leaning forward or backward. In a lunge position, keep your front knee stacked over your front ankle, rather than allowing it to drop inwardly. We all tend to fall into the "path of least resistance" for our bodies, and your yoga practice is a wonderful opportunity to begin to notice—and shift—into better postural habits.

BODY ATTUNEMENT. While your yoga practice will stretch and strengthen your muscles, its larger purpose is to help you become more present, awake, and aware. As you practice, check in with the physical sensations you are experiencing and use them to become present and alert. We don't always have a lot of practice listening to our bodies, particularly if we've been taught "no pain, no gain." Listening to your body will help you respect its current limitations while mindfully exploring your own capacity.

BREATHING. Your breath is another powerful tool for remaining present in your practice. By focusing on your breath, you will stay connected with your body while engaging in a powerful healing process that can soothe your nervous system and help relieve stress.

WARMING UP

Warming up involves doing some large, full-body movements that mobilize your joints, increase your blood flow, and prepare your body for the practice. Rather than jumping into the poses, start with some general movements that limber your body in preparation for strengthening. Remember that movement prompts the secretion of synovial fluid, which lubricates your joints.

BREATHING

Although there are many different breathing practices you may explore during your yoga practice, there is no one "right" way to breathe. The most important thing is to remain mindful and attentive to your breath—all the way up to your final pose, Savasana. Your breath should be calm and even, with no sharp stops or starts. If you find yourself tensing or holding your breath, see if you can calm your inhalations and exhalations and make them even. Controlling your breath is a powerful tool for regulating your nervous system. But if you can't easily control your breath, it's usually a sign that you are trying something that is beyond your current experience level. Let your breath give you feedback on how you are doing and be a companion throughout your practice.

COUNTING

Teachers often count aloud to help their students remain in a pose for the same amount of time on both sides. Counting can also help you stay mindful and present while practicing. You may also find it helpful to count each pose internally. My favorite way of counting is to simply count my breaths: As a general rule, I will stay in a standing pose for about five slow breaths on each side and in a stretching pose for about 20 breaths on each side.

COOLING DOWN

The end of the yoga class is often called the cooldown, and it's an opportunity to stretch after you have been active. Cooldown stretches include seated Uttanasana (Forward Fold, see page 64), seated twists, and reclined poses. These poses are a wonderful opportunity to stay longer in a supported position and use the warmth from your practice to develop more flexibility and mobility.

When practicing cooldown poses, keep these tips in mind:

1. Move slowly. Stretching works best when you allow the stretch to happen rather than push. Your nervous system needs time to adjust to the pose.

2. Hold each pose for at least 90 seconds to give your nervous system a chance to recalibrate to the stretch and release.

3. Breathe. Slow down your breath and move into a state of deeper relaxation.

PROPS

Props are supportive tools that make poses more safe, accessible, or challenging. Our bodies come in all shapes and sizes, which changes the accessibility of postures. For example, I have long arms relative to my torso, which means it's easy for me to press my palms flat to the floor while sitting with my legs straight. But someone with a longer torso relative to their arms may need to sit on a block in order to root their hands down.

Some props that we will use in this book include blocks, straps, and bolsters. But don't worry if you don't have these on hand—it's easy to substitute common household items for these props.

Firm Block

A block is usually made of foam, cork, or wood, and it is often used to "raise the floor" to make the pose more accessible. For example, sitting directly on the floor can often be challenging if you have tight hips, and sitting on a block can help make this position easier and more comfortable. I often invite practitioners to use blocks in poses like the standing Uttanasana (Forward Fold, see page 64) to help support the weight of the torso and make it easier to anchor the hands. If you don't have a block, you can use a thick book or any other stable object (can of beans, stool, or chair) for support.

Soft Block

Soft blocks are made of chip foam and are usually thinner than firm blocks. These props are often used to cushion sensitive joints (like the knee) from the floor. They can also be used to give the body better alignment (for example, to put as a thin pillow under the head when lying down). If you don't have a soft block, you can use a firm, small pillow or a folded towel instead.

Strap

Straps are usually made of cotton and have a buckle or loop system to make it easy to adjust their length. Straps are helpful for creating more space. For example, if it feels constricting to interlace your hands behind your back, you may hold on to the strap to give your shoulders more space. Straps are also often used for stretching. In a seated Uttanasana (see page 64), for example, you may loop the strap around your feet and hold it to gain more leverage in staying upright and keeping your spine long. If you don't have a strap, you can easily substitute a scarf or even a necktie.

Bolster

A bolster is a large, firm pillow usually formed into a flat rectangular or cylindrical sausage shape. Bolsters are used for many restorative poses and help support the body in a wide variety of positions. For example, you can lie back on a bolster to support your upper back, chest, and head, which would allow you to rest in a restorative chest opener. If you don't have a bolster, you can substitute a large, firm pillow.

MYTHS & MISTAKES

Myth: You have to be flexible to do yoga.

Many folks think you have to be especially limber to be good at yoga. Not so! While yoga will help you *become* more flexible, you don't have to be able to touch your toes (or even your knees) to get started. In fact, I love having students who are less flexible in my classes because they're the ones who will most deeply benefit from a good stretch.

Myth: Yoga involves contortions.

While some of the images out there depict people looking like contortionists and doing fancy poses, the truth is that most of the yoga poses we practice are far less exotic. Many of the poses we'll explore will look very familiar to you.

Myth: Yoga is a religion.

While yoga is steeped in the great and diverse traditions of Hinduism, the yoga practice can be viewed as a pragmatic tool for mindfulness. The purpose of yoga is to help the practitioner cultivate a friendly and more skillful relationship with their mind. From this viewpoint, yoga has much more in common with meditation than religion.

Mistake: No pain, no gain!

Remember that adage, "No pain, no gain"? When we start practicing yoga, there may be a tendency to treat it like a physical sport and try to get it "right." A better goal is to develop a patient and consistent practice that can support you on your journey to greater functionality, well-being, and health.

Mistake: Go through the motions.

We may be tempted to treat yoga as another task to check off our to-do list. "Grocery shop: check. Dog groomed: check. Yoga practice: check." But I'd encourage you to treat it as a personal mini vacation at a spa. Not only is your yoga practice a wonderful opportunity to develop your physical stamina, coordination, and flexibility, but it is also a time for mindful self-care. By letting your yoga practice be a dedicated space for mindfulness and slowing down, you will reap the mental and physical benefits of the practice.

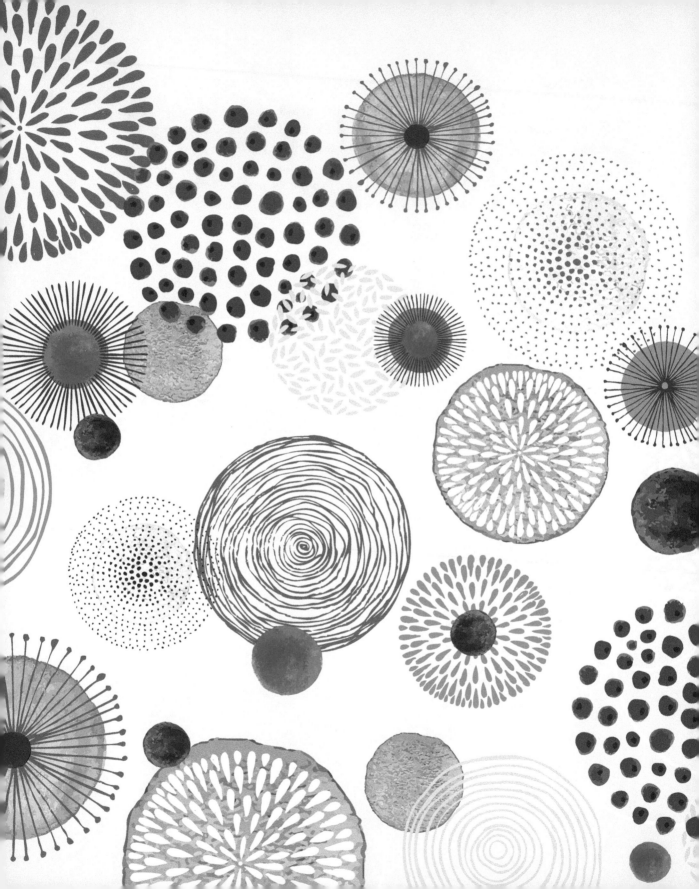

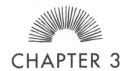

Making It a Personal Practice

EVERYONE IS DIFFERENT

No two bodies are the same.

In the 1950s, the U.S. government embarked on a project to try to improve the design of their cockpits. To create a better design, they measured more than 4,000 pilots and their 140 different bodily dimensions to find out what the "average" pilot looked like. Turned out, creating an average standard was impossible. There's no such thing as an "average" human. Ultimately, the government decided to create the adjustable seats and harnesses that are used today. If we could somehow look at our own skeletons, we would see that each of us has differently shaped bones and joints. And while the average number of bones in the human body is 206, many people have fewer or more bones. The intrinsic differences between our bodies mean that no one's yoga pose will be exactly the same as someone else's.

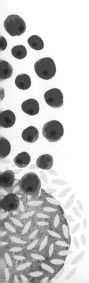

When practicing yoga, seek to cultivate "optimal" rather than "perfect" alignment. Your "optimal" alignment is simply your best at that point in time. Your capacity can change radically over time (and even from day to day), so it's important to listen to your body whenever you arrive on the mat. Treat every practice as a fresh opportunity to ask, "How do I feel today?"

YOGA AT EVERY STAGE OF LIFE

Movement is medicine. Because yoga is so adaptable, the practice can be modified for any stage of life. Whether you are practicing powerful sun salutations to work up a sweat or cultivating mindful mobility through a supported chair practice, yoga will support your health and wellness at any age. As one of my teachers said, "If you can breathe, you can do yoga!"

In our twenties, we are at our peak capacity for physical fitness. We naturally have good muscle mass, higher metabolisms, and healthy cells. However, muscle loss (sarcopenia) can begin to affect people as early as their thirties.

During this time, it's important to keep active in order to develop the positive physical fitness regimes and habits that can sustain us as we grow older. Making yoga a part of our overall plan for healthcare can set us up for future success.

As we move into our forties and fifties, our metabolism slows, and the body tends to recover from injury more slowly. Although we still may be strong, we may begin to see some of the wear and tear that comes from walking around on the planet for a few decades. Bad postural habits may cause chronic tightness in our bodies or add stress to our spines. Women moving into menopause may begin to lose bone density, which can be countered with resistance training. Although we don't use weights in yoga, we are continually supporting our own body weight, which can be helpful in keeping bones strong.

In our sixties, muscle mass tends to decrease, and wear and tear on the spine may lead to disc degeneration or other spinal issues. Physical exercise can help both the body and mind stay vibrant. Yoga's emphasis on spinal health and alignment can help bring mindfulness to daily postural habits.

Entering our seventies and beyond, mitochondrial aging may impact muscular regeneration (mitochondria are organelles inside our cells that help convert sugar to the energy; as we age, they become dysfunctional), making it more challenging to maintain muscle mass. Joint hydration and mobility may decrease, and joint degeneration may lead to arthritis and inflammation. During this time, a low-impact practice like yoga can help maintain joint mobility without putting undue pressure on sensitive joints.

Although many different factors cause the loss of muscle tissue, research shows that exercise and weight-bearing activities can help prevent that loss and slow other markers of aging. And physical exercise and movement help mobilize our joints as well as increase blood and lymph flow, which is beneficial at any stage of life.

YOGA AT DIFFERENT TIMES OF DAY

Although yoga is traditionally practiced in the very early morning, you can practice it at any time of day. The right hour is whenever it works to get your mat! However, it's important to be aware that your body may feel different depending on the time you are practicing.

In the morning, you may feel stiffer during your yoga practice because the intervertebral discs of the spine plump up with water at night. Joints also tend to be a little less mobile in the morning, as they probably haven't been moving much during sleep. So, a flowing yoga practice with large body movements can help wake up the joints and bring some modest movements to the spine.

Around noon, your joints and muscles have likely been warmed up by daily movement, and it may feel appropriate to do a stronger, strength-building practice. If your body is naturally more mobile at this time, you could consider doing a more active practice that helps sustain your energy.

Practicing in the evening can be a nourishing way to unwind from your day and prepare your body and mind for sleep. After a day of activity, long holds and deeper stretches will feel good and help release habitual tightness and sore muscles. Slowing down your practice and doing reclined poses will pacify the nervous system and set you up for deep rest.

CUSTOMIZE YOUR ROUTINE

What you need from your practice can change from day to day and even moment to moment. Use the "Change It Up" tips in part 2 to modify your poses as need. You can dial up the intensity when you want to add more fire and build more strength, or dial it back when you need to rest. Refer to chapter 14 on page 191 to create your own customized yoga routine.

CONSIDER YOUR OPTIONS

Although we often start our yoga journey by learning the physical poses, there is so much more to yoga than the postures. As you cultivate your practice, explore adding in other elements from the tradition, such as breathing practices, seated or reclined meditation, chanting, or even mantras. If you'd like to learn more about mindfulness and yoga philosophy, there are many wonderful books that you can explore about this remarkable tradition, many of which I've listed in the Resources section (see page 194).

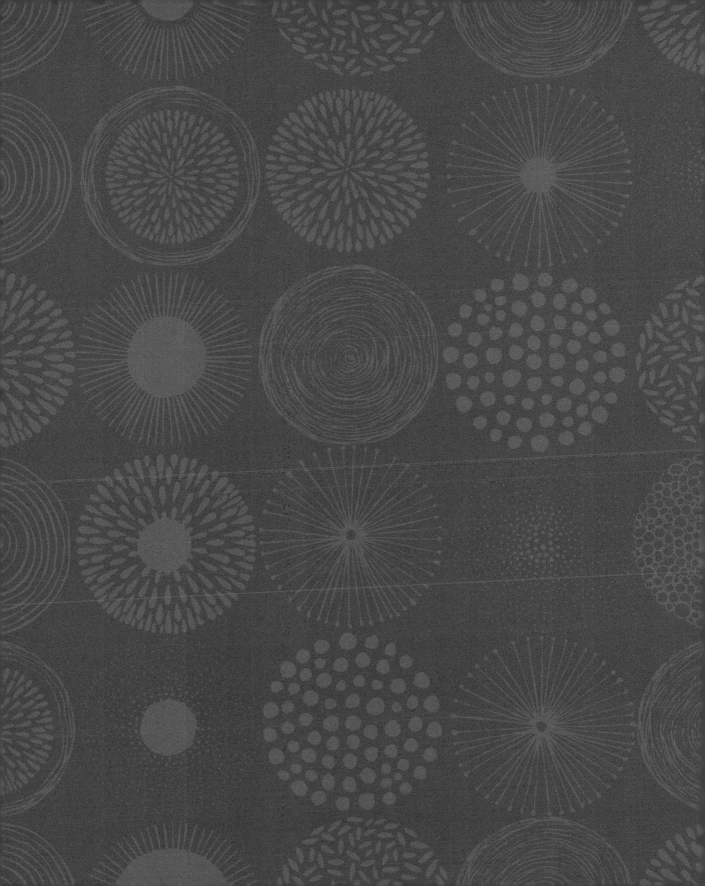

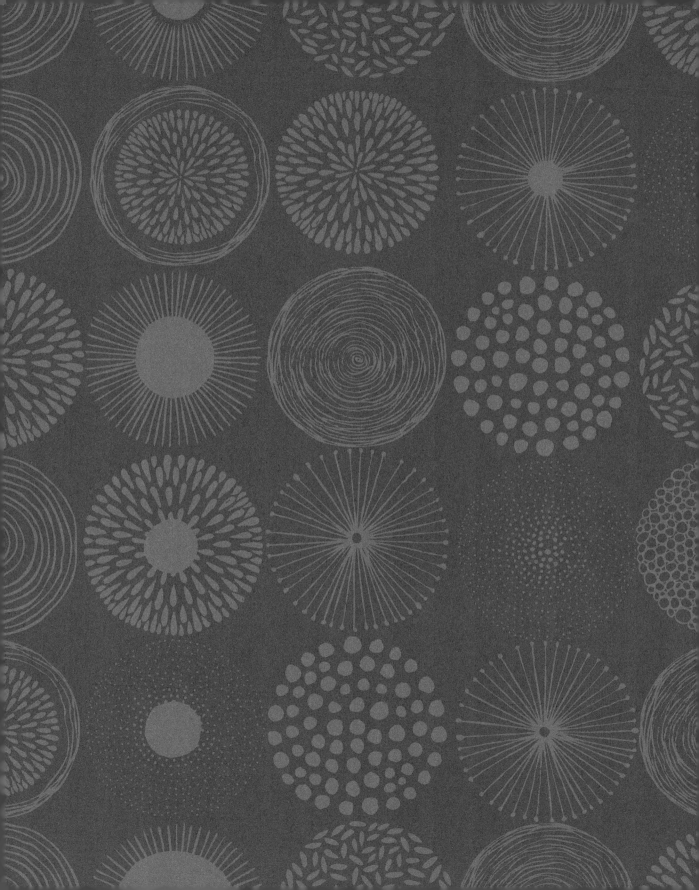

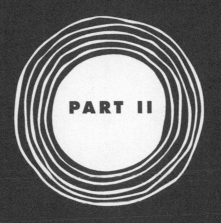

PART II

THE POSES

In the following chapters, you will find a detailed breakdown of the fundamental yoga poses. Each pose description includes an overview of the pose, step-by-step instructions, modifications and variations, and tips for practice. You can do these poses on their own or put them together by following one of the suggested sequences in part 3.

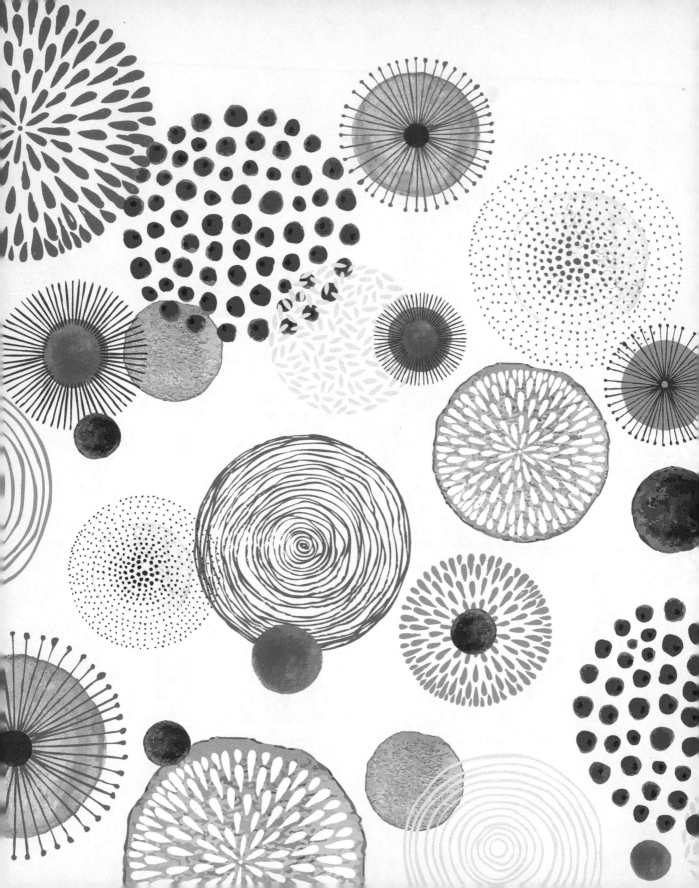

Neck and Shoulders

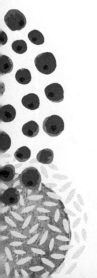

Simple Neck Stretches

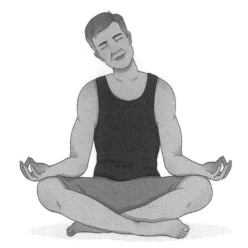

WARM-UP • COOLDOWN • PASSIVE •
PROP: OPTIONAL CHAIR

AFFECTED AREAS

Neck
Superior shoulder muscles

GOOD FOR

✦ Gently releasing tension through the
sides of the neck, throat, and the tops of the shoulders
✦ Stretching the trapezius, levator scapulae, scalenes

INSTRUCTIONS

1. Keeping the chest lifted and open, gently lower your chin toward your chest and take five deep breaths to stretch the back of your neck.
2. Lift your head back upright. Then, move your right ear toward your right shoulder to stretch the left side of your neck. Keep your left shoulder down. Option: Slowly turn your chin down toward your right shoulder, then bring it back to center to adjust the stretch to the side of your neck. Take five deep breaths.
3. Bring your head back upright, then move your ear toward the left shoulder to stretch the right side of your neck. Take five deep breaths. Then lift your head back upright.

CHANGE IT UP

✦ This pose can be performed sitting, seated on a chair, or standing.
✦ Increase the intensity by reaching with your opposite fingertips (for example, if your head is tilted to the right, reach with your left hand).

REMEMBER For the best results, keep your chest open and broad, with your shoulders drawn back and down.

Gomukhasana Arms
(COW FACE POSE, ARMS ONLY)

WARM-UP • COOLDOWN • PASSIVE •
PROP: OPTIONAL CHAIR

AFFECTED AREAS

Back
Shoulders

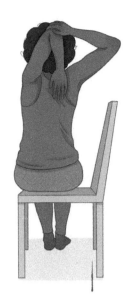

GOOD FOR

+ Improving shoulder mobility
+ Stretching the trapezius, triceps, and latissimus dorsi

INSTRUCTIONS

1. As you inhale, reach your right arm up to the sky.
2. Bend your elbow and place your hand on your back between your shoulder blades.
3. Use your left hand to hold your right elbow in place.
4. Hold for five breaths, then change sides.

CHANGE IT UP

+ This pose can be performed sitting on your mat, seated on a chair, or standing.
+ Decrease the intensity by keeping your hand free (off your back) or allowing it to drift toward the opposite shoulder rather than the middle of the back.
+ Increase the intensity by bringing your hand toward the same shoulder.
+ This arm position can be added to standing poses as a shoulder stretch.
+ Increase the intensity (if you have the shoulder mobility) by taking your left hand back behind your back and reaching up to hold your own fingers.

REMEMBER

- Rather than allowing your ribs to pop forward, keep your lower ribs softening inward.
- To avoid letting the chin drop, keep your chin level with the floor.

Garudasana Arms
(EAGLE POSE, ARMS ONLY)

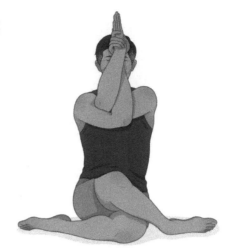

WARM-UP • COOLDOWN • ACTIVE •
PROP: OPTIONAL CHAIR

AFFECTED AREAS

Shoulders
Upper back

GOOD FOR

✦ Improving shoulder mobility
✦ Stretching the back and shoulders

INSTRUCTIONS

1. Inhale and reach your arms wide, parallel to the floor.
2. As you exhale, cross your right arm underneath your left and hold on to your opposite shoulders (like you're giving yourself a hug).
3. If your elbows are crossed, then either press the back of your forearms and hands together, or wind your forearms and press your palms.
4. Hold for five slow, deep breaths.
5. Release and change sides.

CHANGE IT UP

✦ This pose can be performed sitting on your mat, seated on a chair, or standing.
✦ Decrease the intensity by holding your opposite shoulders rather than wrapping your forearms.
✦ This arm position can be added to standing poses such as Virabhadrasana Two (Warrior Two, see page 67) to incorporate a shoulder stretch.

REMEMBER

• Rather than allowing them to lift, drop your shoulders down.
• If your arms are wrapped, lift your elbows and press your hands forward to increase the stretch.

Yoga Mudra
(SEAL POSE)

WARM-UP · COOLDOWN · ACTIVE ·
PROPS: OPTIONAL STRAP OR CHAIR

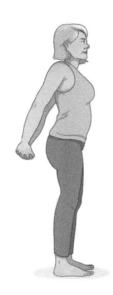

AFFECTED AREAS

Anterior shoulders
Upper chest

GOOD FOR

+ Improving shoulder mobility
+ Opening the upper chest
+ Improving breathing

INSTRUCTIONS

1. Bring your hands behind your back and interlace your fingers (keeping your palms apart).
2. Inhale and roll your shoulders back, then stretch your arms straight behind you.
3. Hold for five slow, deep breaths.
4. Release, change the interlock of your hands, and repeat.

CHANGE IT UP

+ This pose can be performed sitting on the floor, seated sideways on a chair, or standing.
+ To create more space in the pose, hold a strap between your hands about shoulder distance apart behind you with your palms facing forward.
+ Increase the intensity by pressing your palms together.
+ This arm position can be added to standing poses to incorporate a shoulder and chest stretch.

REMEMBER

- Rather than allowing your shoulders to drop forward, bring them back and down.
- Keep your elbows microbent to prevent hyperextension.

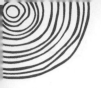

Urdhva Hastasana
(UPWARD HANDS POSE)

WARM-UP · COOLDOWN · ACTIVE ·
PROPS: OPTIONAL STRAP OR CHAIR

AFFECTED AREAS

Back
Neck
Shoulders

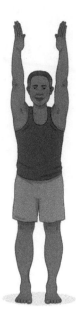

GOOD FOR

✦ Improving shoulder mobility
✦ Stretching the latissimus dorsi, deltoids, and trapezius

INSTRUCTIONS

1. From a seated or standing position, reach your arms straight forward with your palms facing each other. Ensure your arms are straight.
2. Keep your front ribs drawn inward and relax your shoulders away from your ears.
3. Keeping your arms straight and your outer arms squeezing in, reach your arms forward and up toward the sky.
4. Hold for five slow, deep breaths.

CHANGE IT UP

+ This pose can be performed sitting on the floor, seated on a chair, or standing.
+ To create more space in the pose, hold a strap between your hands at least shoulder distance apart with your palms facing forward.
+ Increase the intensity by interlacing your fingers and pressing your palms up toward the sky. Do this variation twice so that you can change the interlock of your fingers.
+ Add a side stretch.
+ This arm position can be added to standing poses to incorporate a shoulder and chest stretch.

REMEMBER

- Rather than allowing your shoulders to hunch or drop forward, keep them lifted and relaxed away from your ears, and also relax the muscles along the sides of your neck.
- Instead of allowing your ribs to pop forward, draw them inward.
- Don't bend your elbows—keep your arms straight (even if it means not lifting your arms as much).

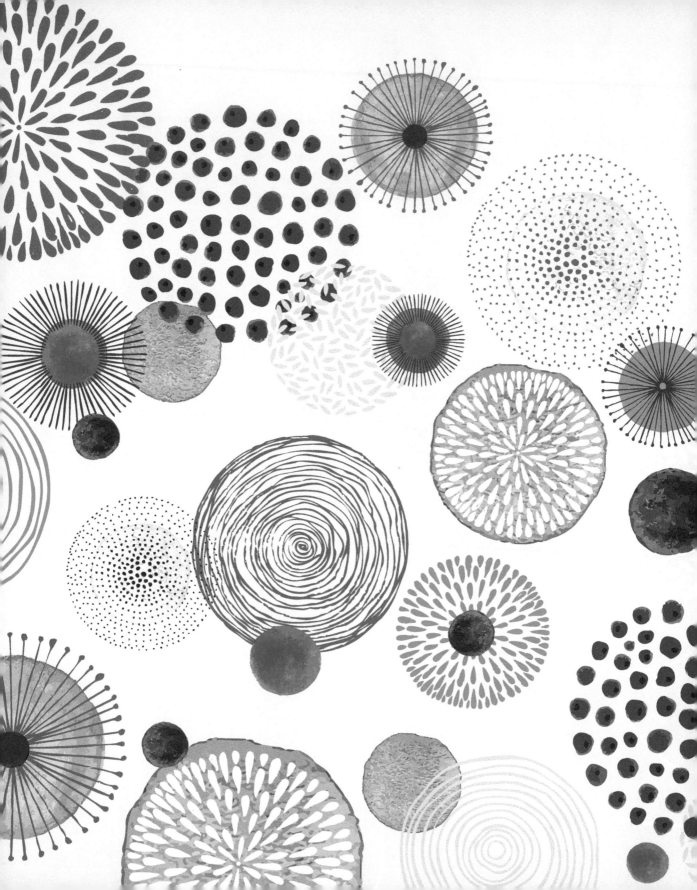

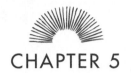

CHAPTER 5

Chest, Back, and Torso

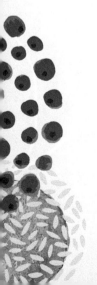

Tadasana
(MOUNTAIN POSE)

....
ACTIVE
PROP: OPTIONAL CHAIR
....

AFFECTED AREAS

Whole body

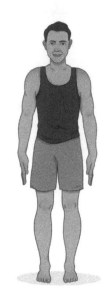

GOOD FOR

+ Strengthening the legs and core
+ Opening the chest and finding proper posture
+ Supporting balance

INSTRUCTIONS

1. Stand with your feet hip distance apart and stack your pelvis, ribs, and head.
2. Root down through the four corners of both feet and spread your toes.
3. Engage your legs (quadriceps and hamstrings) and lift evenly out of all four sides of your waist.
4. Draw your front ribs and your shoulders back.
5. As you lift through your head, stretch your fingers toward the floor by your sides.

CHANGE IT UP

+ Increase your support by sitting in a chair.
+ Add arm variations (interlace your hands behind your back or reach your arms overhead) to add in a shoulder stretch.

REMEMBER

- Although Tadasana may look like you are simply standing, it is an active pose where you work to improve your posture.
- Root strongly down through your feet and lift through the top of your head to find your maximum height.
- Work to find height in your spine by lifting out of your hips and drawing your shoulder blades together.

Savasana
(CORPSE POSE)

....

PASSIVE • COOLDOWN •
PROPS: OPTIONAL BOLSTER,
PILLOW, BLANKET, OR SOCKS

....

AFFECTED AREAS

Whole body

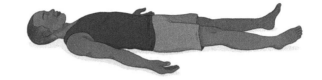

GOOD FOR

✦ Completely resting
✦ Relaxing the nervous system
✦ Integrating the benefits of the practice

INSTRUCTIONS

1. Lie down on your back. If it's uncomfortable to extend the legs, you may keep your knees bent or place a bolster underneath them for support.
2. Rest your arms by your sides with your palms facing up.
3. Close your eyes and completely relax.

CHANGE IT UP

✦ Support your low back by placing a bolster under your knees or putting your calves on a chair or the couch.
✦ If your chin is tilting up to the sky, place a thin pillow under your head so that the back of your neck is long and your chin is slightly tucked.
✦ Stay warm—place a blanket over your body and put your socks back on.

REMEMBER

• Savasana is the last pose in many yoga sequences and is considered an essential component of the practice. Plan to rest in the pose for at least five minutes to reset your nervous system and let your body absorb the benefits of the practice.
• Let your body weight be completely supported by the floor.
• Allow your breath to be natural and easy.
• It's okay to fall asleep!

Spinal Stretch at the Wall

WARM-UP · COOLDOWN · ACTIVE ·
PROP: WALL

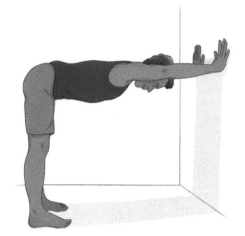

AFFECTED AREAS

Hamstrings
Hands
Shoulders
Spine

GOOD FOR

✦   Opening the shoulders
✦   Stretching the wrists and hands, spine,
    and hamstrings

INSTRUCTIONS

1.   Place your hands on the wall at hip height and outer shoulder distance apart.
2.   Walk your feet back until they're are under your hips and you are in a L-shape.
3.   Bend your knees to pull your hips back.
4.   Press into your hands evenly and squeeze your outer arms in.
5.   Hold for five to 10 breaths.

CHANGE IT UP

✦   Decrease the intensity by bending your elbows slightly and squeezing them in.
✦   Increase the intensity by lifting one foot off the floor and stretching the
    heel back.

REMEMBER

·   Stay rooted through your hands and keep your arms strong and straight.
·   Keep your head aligned with your upper arms rather than dropping it.
·   Rather than rounding or collapsing your spine, keep it long and even.

Balasana
(CHILD'S POSE)

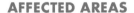

PASSIVE • COOLDOWN •
PROPS: OPTIONAL BLANKET
OR PILLOW

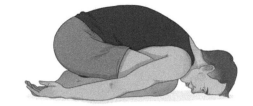

AFFECTED AREAS

Ankles

Feet

Low back

GOOD FOR

✦   Stretching the low back
✦   Resting in the practice

INSTRUCTIONS

1.   Kneel with your knees hip distance apart and your toes together.
2.   Exhale and send your hips back to your heels and bring your belly to your thighs.
3.   Rest your head on a support on the floor, and let your arms rest where they are comfortable (by your sides or head).

CHANGE IT UP

✦   Make this an active pose: Reach your arms forward, keep your hands shoulder distance apart, press your hands firmly down, actively straighten both arms, and reach your fingertips away from your hips.
✦   Add support by placing a blanket or pillow between your shins and thighs, and between your thighs and chest.

REMEMBER

•   Balasana is usually considered a resting pose and is available to you at any time if you need to take a break.
•   If your ankles are uncomfortable, place a rolled-up towel between the front of your ankle and the floor for support.

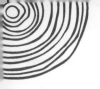

Bhujangasana

(COBRA POSE)

....

ACTIVE

....

AFFECTED AREAS

Back

Chest

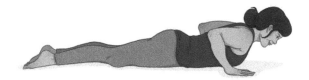

GOOD FOR

✦ Strengthening the spinal extensors
and muscles of the upper back

✦ Stretching the chest

INSTRUCTIONS

1. On your mat, lie prone on your belly with your legs straight and neutral so they aren't turning out—keep your inner thighs rolling up toward the ceiling so the tops of your feet are flat.
2. Place your palms flat under your shoulders.
3. Keeping your legs straight and neutral, lengthen your tailbone to your heels to engage your core and support your lumbar spine.
4. Inhale and lift your upper chest off the floor. Squeeze your shoulder blades toward each other.
5. Hold for five slow, deep breaths.

CHANGE IT UP

✦ Increase or decrease the intensity of the pose by moderating how much you lift your chest.

✦ To increase the load on your back muscles, lift your hands off the floor.

✦ To create more space across the front of your chest, move your hands wide (off your mat) and "stand" your fingers below your elbows (this variation is called "Fingerstand Cobra").

REMEMBER

- Rather than allowing your shoulders to drop forward, keep your shoulders relaxed away from your ears.
- To avoid lifting your chin, look down slightly and keep the back of your neck long.
- Focus the backbend into your upper back by squeezing your shoulder blades together.
- If you feel any sharp compression in your low back, lower your chest until you feel comfortable.

Salabhasana
(LOCUST POSE)

ACTIVE
PROP: OPTIONAL STRAP

AFFECTED AREAS

Back

Chest

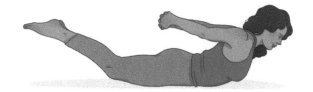

GOOD FOR

✦ Strengthening the spinal extensors, glutes, and hamstrings
✦ Stretching the chest

INSTRUCTIONS

1. On your mat, lie prone on your belly with your legs straight and neutral so they aren't turning out—keep your inner thighs rolling up toward the ceiling.
2. Interlace your hands behind your back.
3. Keeping your legs straight and neutral, lengthen your tailbone to your heels to engage your core and support the lumbar spine.
4. Inhale and lift your chest and legs off the floor. Reach your hands back toward your heels to lift your chest.
5. Hold for five slow, deep breaths.

CHANGE IT UP

✦ To create more space in the pose, hold a strap between your hands at least shoulder distance apart with your palms facing down, or allow your arms to be free.
✦ Decrease the intensity of the pose by keeping your legs on the floor or lifting one leg at a time.
✦ To increase the load on your back muscles, reach your arms forward (this variation is called the Superman Pose).

REMEMBER

- Rather than allowing your shoulders to drop forward, keep them relaxed away from your ears.
- Instead of lifting your chin, look down slightly and keep the back of your neck long.
- Focus the backbend into your upper back by squeezing your shoulder blades together.
- If you feel any sharp compression in your low back, lower your legs or don't lift them up as high.

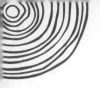

Sphinx Pose

ACTIVE

AFFECTED AREAS

Back
Chest

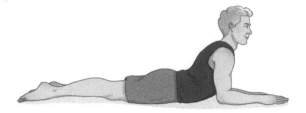

GOOD FOR

✦ Strengthening the spinal extensors
✦ Stretching the chest

INSTRUCTIONS

1. On your mat, lie prone on your belly with your legs straight and neutral so they aren't turning out—keep your inner thighs rolling up toward the ceiling.
2. Prop yourself up on your forearms so that your elbows are directly below your shoulders and your forearms are parallel in front of you.
3. Keeping your legs straight and neutral, lengthen your tailbone to your heels to engage your core and support the lumbar spine.
4. Inhale and press your forearms and hands down to pull your chest forward and open.
5. Hold for five slow, deep breaths.

CHANGE IT UP

✦ To create more space for your low back in the pose, walk your forearms forward so that your lower ribs stay connected to the floor and your low back stays long.
✦ To increase the backbend and load on your arms, lift your elbows off the floor and begin to straighten your arms.

REMEMBER

- Rather than allowing your shoulders to drop forward, keep your shoulders relaxed back and down.
- Instead of lifting your chin, look down slightly and keep the back of your neck long.
- Focus the backbend into your upper back by squeezing your shoulder blades together.
- If you feel any sharp compression in your low back, move your elbows forward to create more space for your back.

Ustrasana
(CAMEL POSE)

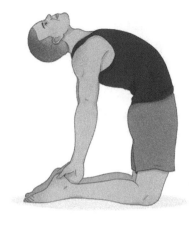

ACTIVE
PROPS: OPTIONAL BLANKET OR CHAIR

AFFECTED AREAS

Back
Chest
Core

GOOD FOR

+ Strengthening the core and upper back
+ Stretching the chest

INSTRUCTIONS

1. Kneel on your mat with your knees hip distance apart and your shins parallel, keeping your toes tucked under your shins. If needed, place a blanket under your knees for cushioning.
2. Place your hands on your hips and draw your elbows back.
3. Root strongly through your shins, lift your chest, and squeeze your shoulder blades together.
4. Inhale, reach your hands to your heels, and lift your chest to the sky.
5. Hold for five slow, deep breaths.

CHANGE IT UP

+ Decrease the intensity of the pose by leaving your hands on your hips.
+ Increase the intensity of the backbend by flattening your feet rather than tucking your toes.
+ Supported Ustrasana in chair: Sitting in your chair, find a seated backbend by holding the chair seat, drawing the shoulders back, and strongly lifting your chest forward and up.

REMEMBER

- Rather than collapsing your back, actively lift your chest forward and up.
- Instead of dropping your head back, tuck your chin slightly to keep the back of your neck long.
- Focus the backbend into your upper back by squeezing your shoulder blades together.
- If you feel any sharp compression in your low back, opt for a more supported backbend like Salabhasana (see page 44), Bhujangasana (see page 42), or Sphinx Pose (see page 46).

Cat/Cow Pose

ACTIVE
PROPS: OPTIONAL BLANKET OR CHAIR

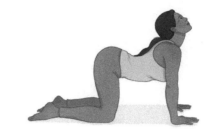

AFFECTED AREAS

Back
Chest
Core
Spine

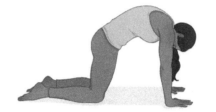

GOOD FOR

✦   Mobilizing the spine

INSTRUCTIONS

1. Start on all fours in a tabletop position with your knees under your hips and your hands shoulder distance apart. Toes may be tucked or untucked.
2. Inhale, release your belly to the floor, and send your tailbone up and back as you reach your chest forward (like a cow).
3. Exhale and arch your spine to the ceiling (like a cat).
4. Repeat five to 10 times.

CHANGE IT UP

✦   Decrease the intensity and increase your support by doing a seated Cat/Cow Pose: Put your hands on your thighs, inhale to open your chest (mini back-bend), and exhale to arch your spine.
✦   Increase the intensity of the pose by reaching your leg back on the inhale or by reaching your opposite hand forward ("dancing" Cat/Cow Pose).

REMEMBER
- Match your movements to your breath.
- Stay rooted through your hands.

Setu Bandha Sarvangasana
(BRIDGE POSE)

ACTIVE
PROP: OPTIONAL BLOCK

AFFECTED AREAS

Back
Chest
Glutes
Hamstrings

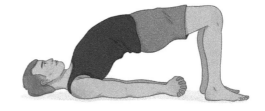

GOOD FOR

✦ Strengthening the glutes, spinal extensors, and chest

INSTRUCTIONS

1. Lie on your back with your knees bent and your feet under your knees.
2. Make "robot arms" by bending at your elbows so that your fingers point straight up to the sky and your upper arms can root down.
3. Root strongly through your feet and lift your hips.
4. Press your upper arms down, widen your collarbone, and lift your chest.
5. Hold for five slow, deep breaths.

CHANGE IT UP

✦ Decrease the intensity of the pose by making it restorative: Put a block or book under your hips to support the weight of your pelvis.
✦ Increase intensity by holding the edges of your mat with your hands (or inter-lacing your hands under your back) and lifting your chest up to your chin.

REMEMBER

• Keep your head relaxed on the floor and your legs parallel.
• Root strongly into your heels and imagine dragging them toward you to lengthen the low back.
• Squeeze your shoulder blades together to lift your chest.

Ardha Matsyendrasana
(SEATED TWIST)

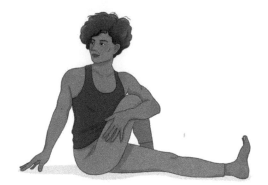

ACTIVE
PROPS: OPTIONAL BLOCK, BOLSTER,
BLANKET, OR CHAIR

AFFECTED AREA

Spine

GOOD FOR

✦   Spinal mobility
✦   Strengthening the muscles along the spine

INSTRUCTIONS

1.   Sit on the floor with your legs straight in front of you.
2.   With your sitting bones evenly rooted, bend your right knee and place your right foot to the outside of your left knee.
3.   Inhale, lift your left arm, and bring your right fingertips behind you.
4.   Exhale, wrap your left arm around your right knee, and twist to the right.
5.   Hold for five slow, deep breaths. Change sides.

CHANGE IT UP

+ If your spine is arched, lift your hips higher by sitting on a block, bolster, or blanket.
+ Rather than sitting on the floor, sit on a chair with your feet flat on the floor. You can hold the chair back to help you twist.
+ Increase the intensity of the twist by bringing your left elbow to the outside of your knee.
+ If it feels appropriate for your knee and you can keep your sitting bones grounded, bend your left leg and bring your left heel to the outside of your right hip.

REMEMBER

- Inhale to lengthen, exhale to twist.
- Keep your chest open and broad.
- Hold your pelvis stable and your sitting bones evenly rooted into the prop or floor.

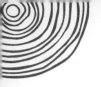

Parivrtta Parsvakonasana
(REVOLVED LOW OR HIGH LUNGE)

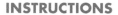

ACTIVE
PROP: OPTIONAL CUSHION
FOR BACK KNEE

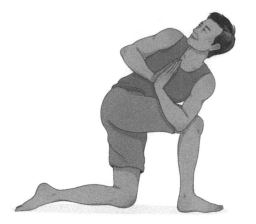

AFFECTED AREA

Spine

GOOD FOR

+ Spinal mobility
+ Strengthening the muscles along
  the spine
+ Balance

INSTRUCTIONS

1. From an Uttanasana (Forward Fold position, see page 64) position at the front of
   your mat, step your left foot back and lower your back knee so that you are in a
   low lunge position (option: use a cushion to support your knee).
2. Bring your hands onto your front thigh.
3. Inhale and lift your left arm.
4. Exhale and place your elbow outside your right knee; press your palms together
   and twist your spine to the right.
5. Hold for five slow, deep breaths. Change sides.

CHANGE IT UP

+ Decrease the intensity of the pose by placing your hand (rather than elbow)
  outside your knee and your top hand on your hip.
+ Increase the intensity of the pose by lifting your back knee off the floor.

REMEMBER

• Inhale to lengthen, exhale to twist.
• Keep your pelvis stable and your sitting bones evenly rooted.

Parivrtta Utkatasana
(REVOLVED CHAIR POSE)

ACTIVE
PROP: OPTIONAL CHAIR

AFFECTED AREA

Spine

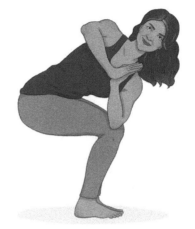

GOOD FOR

- ✦ Spinal mobility
- ✦ Strengthening the muscles along the spine

INSTRUCTIONS

1. Stand at the front of your mat with your feet together. Bend your knees and send your hips back and down to sit into a chair position.
2. Inhale and lengthen your spine.
3. Exhale and place your elbow outside your right knee; press your palms together, and twist your spine to the right.
4. Hold for five slow, deep breaths. Change sides.

CHANGE IT UP

- ✦ Decrease the intensity of the pose by placing your hand (rather than elbow) outside your knee and your top hand on your hip.
- ✦ Increase the intensity of the pose by sitting lower into the chair position.

REMEMBER

- • Inhale to lengthen, exhale to twist.
- • Keep your chest open and broad.
- • Hold your pelvis stable and your knees aligned.

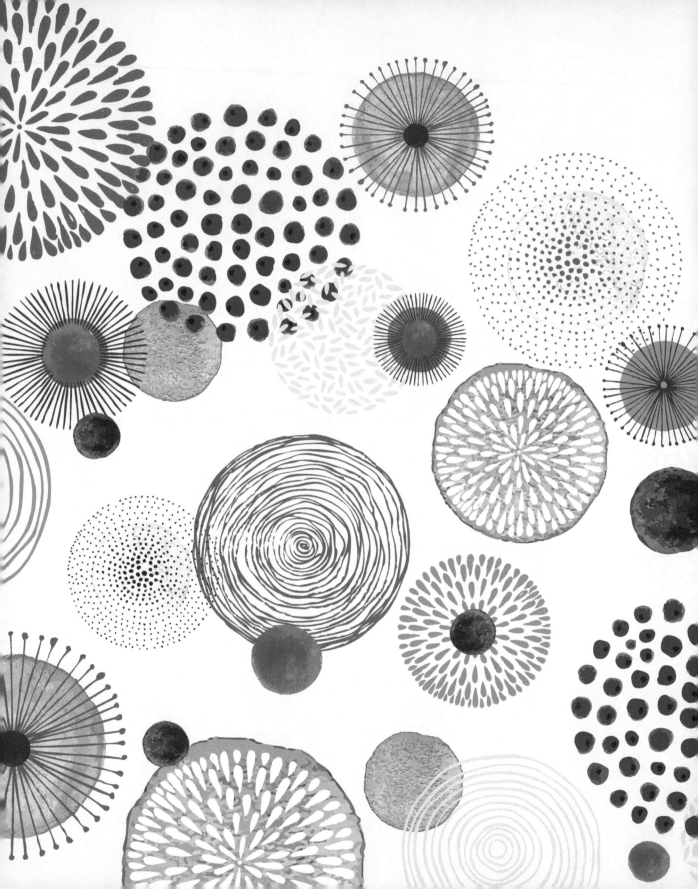

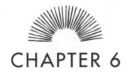

Arms, Wrists, and Hands

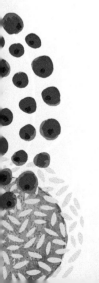

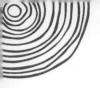

Phalakasana
(PLANK POSE)

ACTIVE • WARM-UP

AFFECTED AREAS

Core
Hands
Wrists

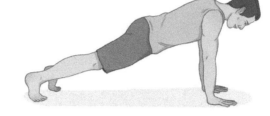

GOOD FOR

✦ Strengthening the arms and core

INSTRUCTIONS

1. Start on all fours in a tabletop position with your knees under your hips and your hands shoulder distance apart.
2. Step your feet back to come into a high push-up position (Plank) with your hips level with your shoulders.
3. Spread your fingers apart and root all four corners of your hands down.
4. Hold for 10 breaths.

CHANGE IT UP

✦ Decrease the intensity of the pose by lowering your knees down.
✦ Also decrease the intensity on your wrists by coming onto your forearms, fists, or even on your fingertips.
✦ Increase the intensity of the pose by lifting one foot at a time.

REMEMBER

• Press your hands down and straighten your arms to keep your chest lifted and spine long.
• Engage your legs and lift your pelvis to keep your hips buoyant and aligned with your shoulders.
• Root through the base of your index knuckle and fingertips to keep the pressure evenly distributed through your hands.

Vasisthasana
(SIDE PLANK POSE)

ACTIVE · WARM-UP

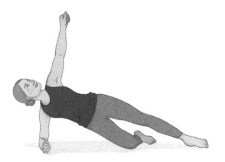

AFFECTED AREAS

Core
Shoulders

GOOD FOR

✦ Strengthening the arms, back, and core
(particularly the obliques)

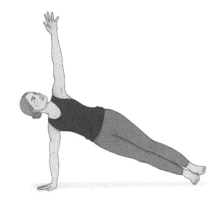

INSTRUCTIONS

1. Come into Phalakasana (Plank Pose, see
page 58) on your forearms with your
hands clasped.
2. Keep your chest lifted, roll onto the outer
edge of your right foot, and stack your feet.
3. Bring your left hand off the floor and to your hip, or lift it.
4. Lift your hips up strongly for two to three breaths, then lower your left elbow.
Take a break, then change sides.

CHANGE IT UP

✦ Increase your support by offsetting your feet rather than stacking them or
bending the top knee and placing the top foot flat on the floor.
✦ Decrease the intensity of the pose by keeping your top hand on the floor rather
than lifting it.
✦ Increase the intensity of the pose by lifting your top foot off the bottom foot.

REMEMBER

• Keep your chest wide as you squeeze your shoulder blades toward
each other.
• Lift your hips as high as you can.

Wrist Stretch

WARM-UP • COOLDOWN • PASSIVE •
PROP: OPTIONAL CHAIR

AFFECTED AREAS

Hands
Wrists

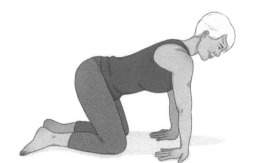

GOOD FOR

✦ Stretching the wrists and forearms

INSTRUCTIONS

1. Start on all fours on your mat.
2. Turn one hand around, palm down, so that your fingers are pointing back toward your body.
3. Stay for five breaths to gently stretch the back of your wrist, then change sides.

CHANGE IT UP

✦ This pose can be performed sitting on your mat, seated on a chair, or standing. Practice it in a chair by extending your right hand forward with your palm forward and fingers pointing down, then using your left hand to gently pull your fingers down.

✦ Increase the intensity of the stretch by drawing your weight back or doing both hands at the same time.

REMEMBER

• Keep the fingers spread wide and the fingertips down.
• Move slowly and gently.

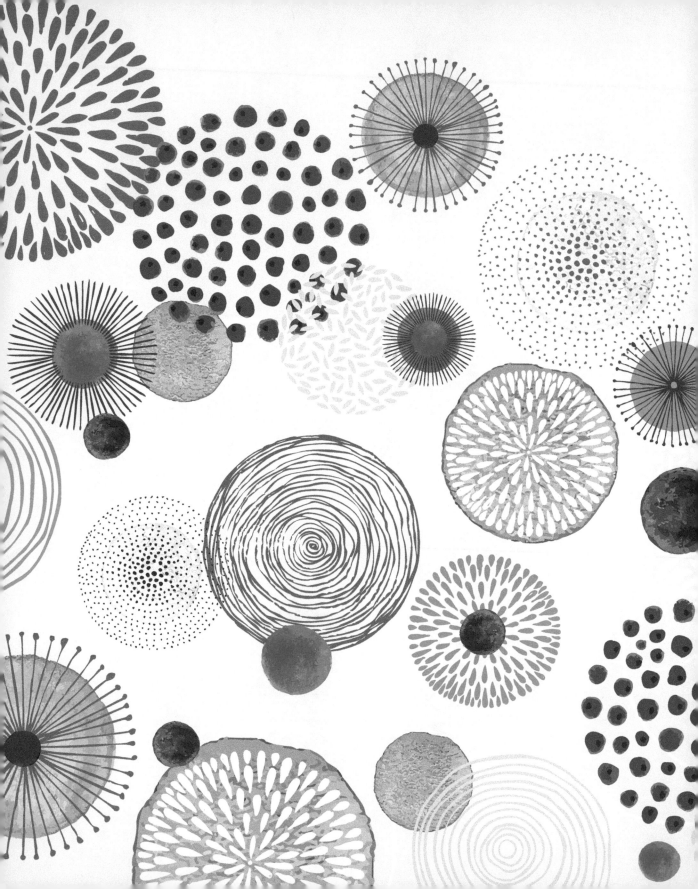

Hips, Buttocks, Thighs, and Hamstrings

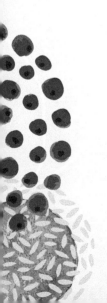

Uttanasana
(FORWARD FOLD)

WARM-UP • PASSIVE •
PROP: OPTIONAL BLOCK OR CHAIR

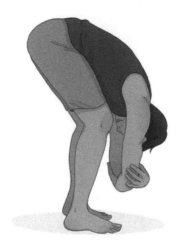

AFFECTED AREAS

Hamstrings (stretching)
Spine (lengthening)

GOOD FOR

✦ Stretching the hamstrings
✦ Releasing the spine

INSTRUCTIONS

1. Stand with your feet hip distance apart and parallel.
2. With your knees slightly bent, hinge forward from your hips and fold over your legs.
3. Hold on to opposite elbows and allow the weight of your upper body to fall to the floor.
4. Slowly work to straighten your legs.
5. After five breaths, change the crossing of your elbows. Stay for five more breaths.
6. Bend your knees slightly and lengthen your spine to come up.

CHANGE IT UP

✦ Make the pose more accessible by placing your hands on blocks or a chair for support and only coming halfway down.
✦ Increase the intensity of the pose by changing the arm variation: Bring your fingertips to the floor, interlace your fingers behind your back, hold on to your big toes, or slide your hands under your feet.

REMEMBER

• Rather than arching your spine, keep it as long as possible and hinge forward from the hips.
• Keep a slight bend in your knees as you engage your quads.

Adho Mukha Svanasana
(DOWNWARD FACING DOG)

WARM-UP · ACTIVE

AFFECTED AREAS

Arms (strengthening)
Calves
Feet
Hamstrings (stretching)
Shoulders (opening)
Spine

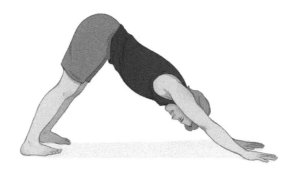

GOOD FOR

✦   Strengthening the upper body
✦   Opening the hamstrings and calves
✦   Stretching the spine

INSTRUCTIONS

1.   Start on your mat on all fours with your hands outer shoulder distance apart and your knees about a foot behind your hips.
2.   Press into your hands, lifting your hips up and back to come into Adho Mukha Svanasana (Downward Facing Dog).
3.   Bend your knees, straighten your arms, and lengthen your spine.
4.   As you lift strongly through your legs, bend one knee and sink the opposite heel to the floor. Hold for five to 10 breaths, then change sides.

CHANGE IT UP

✦   Increase the intensity of the pose by pressing the balls of the feet firmly down. Without actually moving your feet, attempt to scrub—or slide—the balls of your feet back toward the mat as you sink your heels down.
✦   Decrease the intensity of your body weight by lowering your knees down to the floor so that they are below your hips and focusing on stretching the spine.
✦   Increase the intensity of the pose by lifting one foot, then the other, off the floor.

CONTINUED

REMEMBER

- Bend your knees first to lengthen your spine, then work to straighten your legs.
- Press into your inner hands as you hug your outer arms toward each other and straighten your arms.
- Relax your neck.

Virabhadrasana Two
(WARRIOR TWO POSE)

WARM-UP • ACTIVE •
PROP: OPTIONAL CHAIR

AFFECTED AREAS

Gluteus (maximus, medius, and minimus)
Hamstrings (strengthening)
Quadriceps (strengthening)

GOOD FOR

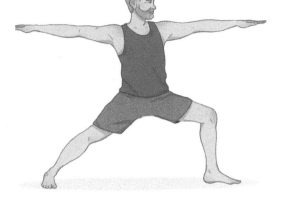

+ Strengthening the legs
+ Improving balance

INSTRUCTIONS

1. Stand facing the broad side of your mat with your feet spread wide apart.
2. Turn your right thigh out so that your foot, shin, knee, and thigh face the short end of your mat and your front heel bisects the arch of your back foot. Turn your back heel out slightly.
3. Bend your front knee to a square with your knee over your ankle.
4. Reach your arms wide and look at your front hand.
5. Hold for five to 10 breaths.

CHANGE IT UP

+ Make the pose more accessible by holding onto a chair for balance or by placing your front thigh on a chair for support (this can also be a great workout for the front thigh).
+ Add a side stretch by reaching your front arm up to the sky as you place your back hand on your back thigh.

REMEMBER

• Keep your front knee bent deeply so that it's over your ankle.
• Keep your front knee aligned over your ankle as you turn your hips toward the broad side of the mat to strengthen your outer glutes.

Parsvakonasana
(SIDE ANGLE POSE)

WARM-UP • ACTIVE •
PROPS: OPTIONAL BLOCK OR CHAIR

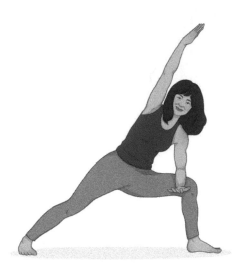

AFFECTED AREAS

Gluteus (maximus, medius, and minimus)
Hamstrings (strengthening)
Quadriceps (strengthening)

GOOD FOR

✦　Strengthening the legs
✦　Improving balance

INSTRUCTIONS

1.　Stand facing the broad side of your mat in Virabhadrasana Two (Warrior Two Pose, see page 67).
2.　Shift your hips toward the back of your mat and place your forearm on your front thigh.
3.　Stretch your top arm up to the sky and widen your chest.
4.　Hold for five to 10 breaths.

CHANGE IT UP

✦　Deepen the pose by placing your bottom hand on a block and moving it to the inside or outside of your front foot.
✦　Increase the intensity of the pose by hovering your front elbow off your thigh.

REMEMBER

· Keep your front knee bent deeply so that it's over your ankle. If your front thigh is not in a square (90 degrees), then consider lengthening your stance.
· Keep your front knee over your ankle as you turn your hips toward the broad side of the mat to strengthen your outer glutes.
· Evenly lengthen both sides of your torso.

Trikonasana
(TRIANGLE POSE)

WARM-UP • ACTIVE •
PROP: BLOCK

AFFECTED AREAS

Gluteus (maximus, medius, and minimus)
Hamstrings (stretching)

GOOD FOR

✦ Strengthening the legs
✦ Stretching the hamstrings
✦ Improving balance

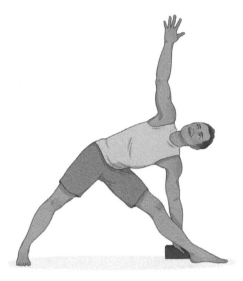

INSTRUCTIONS

1. Stand facing the broad side of your mat in Virabhadrasana Two (Warrior Two Pose, see page 67).
2. Keeping your front thigh rotating open and your knee aligned with your ankle, straighten your front leg.
3. Shift your hips toward the back of your mat and fingertips on a block outside your front shin.
4. Stretch your top arm up to the sky and widen your chest.
5. Hold for five to 10 breaths.

CHANGE IT UP

✦ Decrease the intensity of the stretch by bending your front knee slightly.
✦ Decrease the depth by bringing your fingertips to your shin rather than the block.

REMEMBER

• Keep your outer hip strongly drawing back and under you in order to keep your front foot, shin, knee, and thigh aligned.
• Maintain a microbend in your front knee to prevent hyperextension.

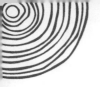

Low Lunge and High Lunge

ACTIVE

PROPS: OPTIONAL CHAIR AND/OR CUSHION FOR BACK KNEE

AFFECTED AREAS

Adductors (strengthening)
Hip flexors (stretching)

GOOD FOR

✦ Opening the hip flexors
✦ Balance

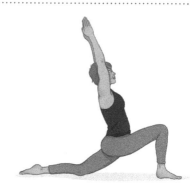
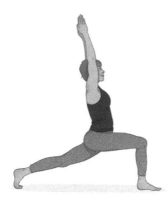

INSTRUCTIONS

1. From an Uttanasana (Forward Fold, see page 64) position at the front of your mat, step your left foot back and lower your back knee so that you are in a low lunge position (option: use a cushion to support your knee).
2. Inhale and reach both arms up.
3. Squeeze your legs together, lengthen your tailbone down, and move your hips forward.
4. Hold for five slow, deep breaths, then change sides.

CHANGE IT UP

✦ Increase the intensity of the pose by lifting your back knee off the floor.
✦ Add a backbend by drawing your upper arms behind your ears and squeezing your shoulder blades together.
✦ Decrease the intensity on your shoulders by bending your elbows into a cactus shape.
✦ Add support by holding onto a chair for balance.

REMEMBER

• Squeeze your inner legs together to keep your hips square.
• Draw your low belly in as you sink your hips forward to increase the hip flexor stretch.
• Squeeze your glute muscles to increase the stability and the stretch.

Utkatasana
(CHAIR POSE)

WARM-UP · ACTIVE · PASSIVE ·
PROP: OPTIONAL CHAIR

AFFECTED AREAS

Glutes
Hamstrings (strengthening)
Quadriceps (strengthening)

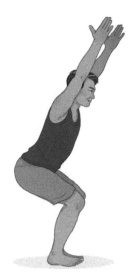

GOOD FOR

✦   Strengthening the legs and glutes

INSTRUCTIONS

1. Stand at the front of your mat with your feet hip distance apart and parallel.
2. Bend your knees and move your hips back and down to sit into a chair position.
3. Keep the muscles at the base of your neck relaxed as you reach your arms forward and up.
4. Hold for five to 10 slow, deep breaths.

CHANGE IT UP

✦   Decrease the intensity in the shoulders by bringing your arms into a cactus position or reaching your arms straight forward.
✦   Increase the intensity of the pose by sitting lower into the chair position.
✦   For added support, sit on the edge of a chair and actively press your feet into the floor.
✦   Add a backbend by drawing your shoulder blades closer together and lifting your chest forward and up.

REMEMBER
·   Lean your weight into your heels and sit down low.
·   Keep your chest open and broad.

Prasarita Padottanasana
(WIDE-LEGGED FORWARD FOLD)

PASSIVE
PROPS: OPTIONAL BLOCKS OR CHAIR

AFFECTED AREA

Hamstrings (stretching)

GOOD FOR

✦ Stretching the hamstrings

INSTRUCTIONS

1. Stand at the front of your mat with your feet wide (about three feet apart) and parallel.
2. Inhale with your hands on your hips, then exhale and hinge from your hips to Uttanasana (Forward Fold, see page 64).
3. Place your fingertips to the floor (or put your hands on blocks).
4. Root into your feet to stretch your legs.
5. Hold for 10 slow, deep breaths.

CHANGE IT UP

✦ Decrease the intensity of the pose by bending your knees.
✦ Increase your support by placing your hands on blocks or a chair.
✦ Add a shoulder stretch by interlacing your hands behind your back and lifting your arms to the sky.

REMEMBER

· Keep your weight even in the front and back of your feet.
· Actively engage your quadriceps to open the hamstrings.
· If it is comfortable, release the weight of your torso and head toward the floor.

Supta Hasta Padangusthasana
(RECLINED LEG STRETCHES)

PASSIVE · COOLDOWN · PROPS: STRAP

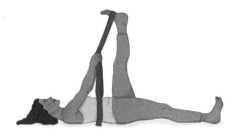

AFFECTED AREAS

Adductors (stretching)
Glutes (stretching)
Hamstrings (stretching)

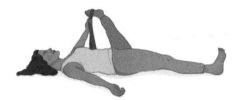

GOOD FOR

✦ Stretching the hamstrings, adductors, and IT band

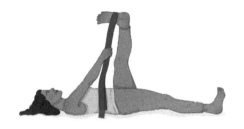

INSTRUCTIONS

1. Lie on your back with your knees bent and your feet under your knees.
2. Place a strap around the ball of your right foot, straighten your right leg, and press your foot to the sky.
3. Stretch 1: Anchor your right hip down and reach your right heel strongly to the sky to stretch your hamstrings. Hold for 10 breaths.
4. Stretch 2: Holding your strap in your right hand, take your right leg wide to the right to stretch the adductors. Hold for 10 breaths.
5. Stretch 3: Keeping your right hip anchored down, hold the strap in your left hand and take your right foot across your body toward your left shoulder to stretch your outer right leg and IT Band. Hold for 10 breaths.
6. Change sides.

CONTINUED

CHANGE IT UP

✦ Decrease the intensity of the stretches by bending your knee.

✦ Increase the intensity of the stretches by extending your left leg straight and pressing your thigh strongly into the mat with your toes pointed straight up to the sky.

✦ To increase your support and avoid tipping over, when you take your leg out to the side (Stretch 2), walk the foot of your bent leg out to the side for counterbalance.

REMEMBER

• Make sure your back and pelvis are firmly and evenly anchored into the floor and keep your pelvis stable through the sequence.
• Keep your chest open and shoulders away from your ears.
• Spread the ball of your foot into the strap.
• Activate the quadriceps to help stretch your leg.

Eka Pada Kapotasana

(PIGEON OR "SLEEPING SWAN" POSE)

PASSIVE • COOLDOWN •
PROPS: OPTIONAL BLOCK

AFFECTED AREA

Glutes (stretching)

GOOD FOR

✦ Stretching the outer hips

INSTRUCTIONS

1. In the middle of your mat, sit on your right hip with your right shin parallel to the front of your mat and your left shin (roughly) parallel to the side of your mat.
2. Uttanasana (Forward Fold, see page 64) over your front knee.
3. Hold for 10 breaths.
4. Change sides.

CHANGE IT UP

✦ Increase the stretch by beginning to straighten your left leg behind you so that your left hip releases toward the floor.
✦ Change the stretch by walking your hands and torso closer to your front foot.
✦ Make the pose more relaxing by resting your head on a block or the floor.

REMEMBER

· The stretching sensation should be in the outer hip, never the knee. If the knee twinges, try "Thread the Needle" pose instead.
· Let your upper body relax as much as possible.

Thread the Needle
(FIGURE FOUR POSE)

PASSIVE • COOLDOWN •
PROPS: OPTIONAL WALL, CHAIR,
STRAP, CUSHION, OR PILLOW

AFFECTED AREA

Glutes (stretching)

GOOD FOR

✦   Stretching the outer hips

INSTRUCTIONS

1. Lie on your back with your knees bent and your feet under your knees.
2. Cross your right ankle over your left knee to make a 90-degree angle in your right leg.
3. Hold on to the back of your left thigh and draw your knee toward your left shoulder.
4. Hold for 10 breaths.
5. Change sides.

CHANGE IT UP

✦   Decrease the intensity of the pose by leaving your left foot on the floor.
✦   Make it passive by doing this pose near the wall, then placing your left foot on the wall (so you don't have to hold it with your hands).
✦   Support the pose by sitting in a chair and crossing your right ankle over your left knee. Hinge forward from your hips.
✦   If you can't easily reach the back of your leg without lifting your chest, use a strap to hold the back of your leg instead.

REMEMBER

· Let your upper body relax as much as possible and your chest stay broad and open. Keep the back of the pelvis anchored down. If your chin is lifting up, place a soft cushion or pillow under your head.
· Breathe into the stretch and exhale to soften.

Ananda Balasana
(HAPPY BABY POSE)

PASSIVE · COOLDOWN ·
PROPS: OPTIONAL CUSHION OR PILLOW

AFFECTED AREA

Adductors (stretching)

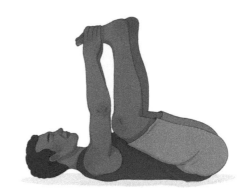

GOOD FOR

✦ Stretching the inner thighs

INSTRUCTIONS

1. Lie on your back and draw your knees into your chest.
2. Take your knees as wide as your chest, then flex your feet and take your shins vertical so that the soles of your feet are toward the sky.
3. Hold on to the backs of your thighs, your shins, or your outer feet to draw the knees toward the outside of your ribs.

CHANGE IT UP

✦ Do one side at a time to move more deeply into each side.
✦ Decrease the intensity of the pose by drawing your knees into your chest, holding the tops of your shins, and allowing your knees to fall wide (keep the shins horizontal rather than vertical).
✦ Roll from side to side like a happy baby on its back.

REMEMBER

• Let your upper body relax as much as possible so that your chest remains broad and open. If your chin is lifting up, place a soft cushion or pillow under your head.
• Breathe into the stretch and exhale to soften.

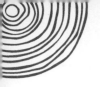

Sukhasana
(EASY SEAT POSE)

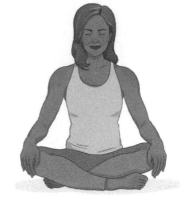

PASSIVE
PROPS: OPTIONAL PILLOW, BOLSTER, BLOCK,
OR CHAIR

AFFECTED AREAS

Outer hips

GOOD FOR

✦ Sitting comfortably to breathe and center yourself at the beginning and end
of practice
✦ Stretching the outer hips when in Uttanasana (Forward Fold, see page 64)

INSTRUCTIONS

1. Sit in a comfortable, cross-legged position with your shins crossed.
2. As you root through your sitting bones, lift your spine upright and draw your
shoulders back.
3. Let your hands rest comfortably on your thighs.

CHANGE IT UP

✦ Change the crossing of your shins to do your non-habitual side.
✦ Add support by sitting on a pillow, bolster, or block.
✦ Add variations by incorporating side stretches or arm poses.
✦ Hinge forward from your hips to create an outer hip stretch, then change the
crossing of your shins and do the other side.

REMEMBER

• In this pose, the spine should be tall and straight. If you find yourself
arching forward or rolling to the back of your sitting bones, sit on a
prop or chair.
• Use this pose to settle into your breath and feel the sensations of
your body.

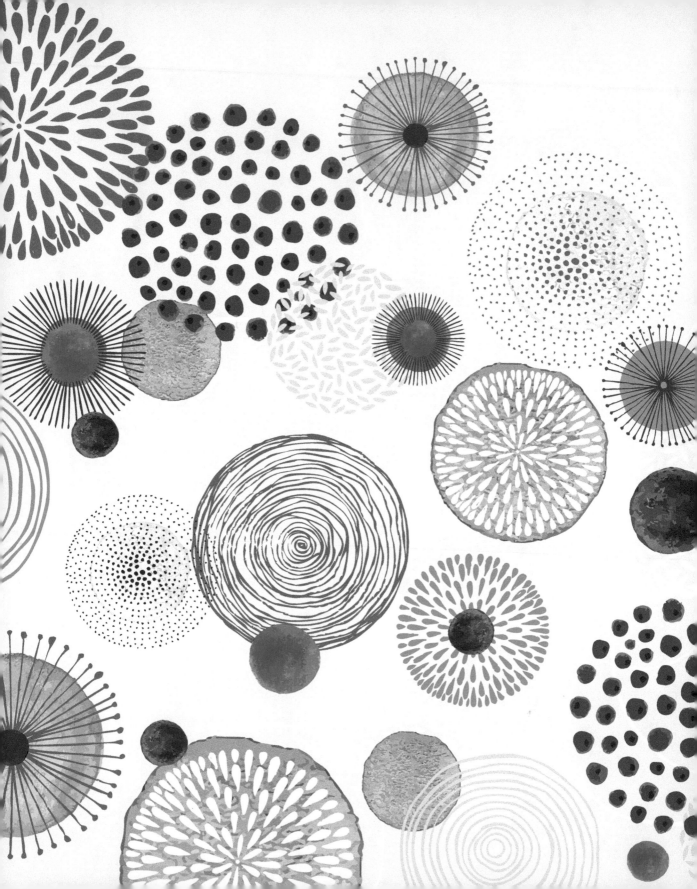

CHAPTER 8

Knees, Calves, and Shins

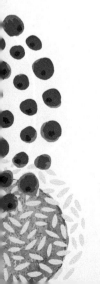

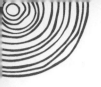

Utkatasana with Heel Lift

WARM-UP • ACTIVE •
PROPS: OPTIONAL WALL OR CHAIR

AFFECTED AREAS

Calves
Feet
Hamstrings
Quadriceps

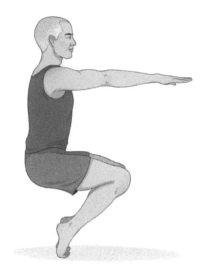

GOOD FOR

✦ Strengthening the legs, glutes, and calves

INSTRUCTIONS

1. Stand at the front of your mat with your feet hip distance apart and parallel. Reach your arms forward (option: touch the wall for support).
2. Lift your heels to balance on the balls of your feet.
3. Keeping your chest lifted, bend your knees, and slide your back down an imaginary wall to come into "Chair Toe Stand."
4. Hold for five slow, deep breaths.

CHANGE IT UP

✦ Decrease the intensity of the pose by keeping your feet flat.
✦ Increase the intensity of the pose by sitting lower into the chair position so that your hips are eventually level with your knees or by slowly lowering down and lifting up three times.
✦ Chair option: Sit in a chair with your feet flat on the floor. Lift your heels and squeeze your calves, holding for five seconds. Repeat 10 times.

REMEMBER

• Lean back and push your knees forward to keep your torso vertical.
• If you feel any pressure in your knees, opt for classic Utkatasana (see page 71) instead.

Virasana
(HERO POSE)

WARM-UP • PASSIVE •
PROPS: BLOCK(S); OPTIONAL CHAIR
OR HAND TOWEL

AFFECTED AREAS

Calves

Feet

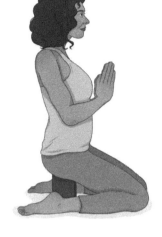

GOOD FOR

✦ Stretching the tops of the feet
✦ Compressing the calves

INSTRUCTIONS

1. Stack one or two blocks lengthwise on your mat.
2. Starting on all fours, bring your feet to either side of your block stack. Point your toes and sit back on the blocks with your thighs parallel.
3. Root your sitting bones down to lift your spine tall and stretch the tops of your feet.
4. Hold for five to 10 slow, deep breaths.

CHANGE IT UP

✦ Increase the intensity of the pose by removing the blocks and sitting with your hips between your feet.
✦ Decrease the intensity of the pose by adding more blocks to sit higher.
✦ Make the pose active: Press your shins firmly into the floor until your hips almost lift off the blocks.
✦ If you feel any pressure in your knees, sit cross-legged or on a chair instead.
✦ If you feel too much pressure in the tops of your feet, place a small rolled-up hand towel under the front of your ankles to lift them away from the floor.

REMEMBER

• Keep your torso vertical and tall.

Modified Virabhadrasana One
(WARRIOR ONE POSE)

WARM-UP • COOLDOWN • PASSIVE •
PROP: WALL

AFFECTED AREAS

Calves

Feet

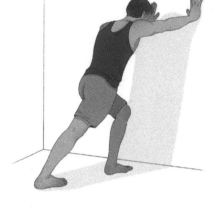

GOOD FOR

✦   Stretching the calves

INSTRUCTIONS

1.   Place your hands on a wall in front of you, step your right foot back about two feet, and perch onto the ball of that foot with your heel up.
2.   Bend your left knee and reach your right heel back and down toward the floor to stretch the back of your calf.
3.   After five to 10 breaths, bend your right knee slightly to access a deeper calf stretch.
4.   Hold for five to 10 breaths, then change sides.

CHANGE IT UP

✦   Increase the intensity of the pose by lengthening your stance.
✦   Test your balance by reaching your arms up to the sky.

REMEMBER

·   Keep your torso vertical and tall.
·   Press your hands into the wall to put more weight on your back heel.

Malasana
(SQUAT OR GARLAND POSE)

COOLDOWN • PASSIVE •
PROPS: OPTIONAL BLOCK

AFFECTED AREAS

Adductors (stretching)
Calves
Feet

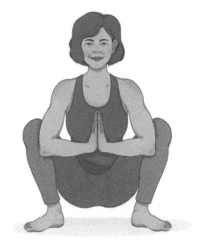

GOOD FOR

✦ Stretching the calves
✦ Stretching the adductors

INSTRUCTIONS

1. Stand with your feet wide apart. Keep your feet at 45-degree angles.
2. Keep your knees tracking over the center of your feet as you bend your knees and lower your hips into a squat.
3. Bring your elbows inside your knees and press your knees wide as you lift your chest. Do your best to anchor your heels down.
4. Hold for five to 10 breaths.

CHANGE IT UP

✦ Increase your support and decrease the intensity on your knees by stopping halfway down and bringing your elbows onto your thighs.
✦ If your heels lift off the floor, increase support by placing them on thin blocks or books of the same size.

REMEMBER

• If you feel any sensation in your knees, use the football coach position.
• Keep your knees, shins, and feet aligned.
• Squeeze your knees into your arms and press your knees wide with your elbows.

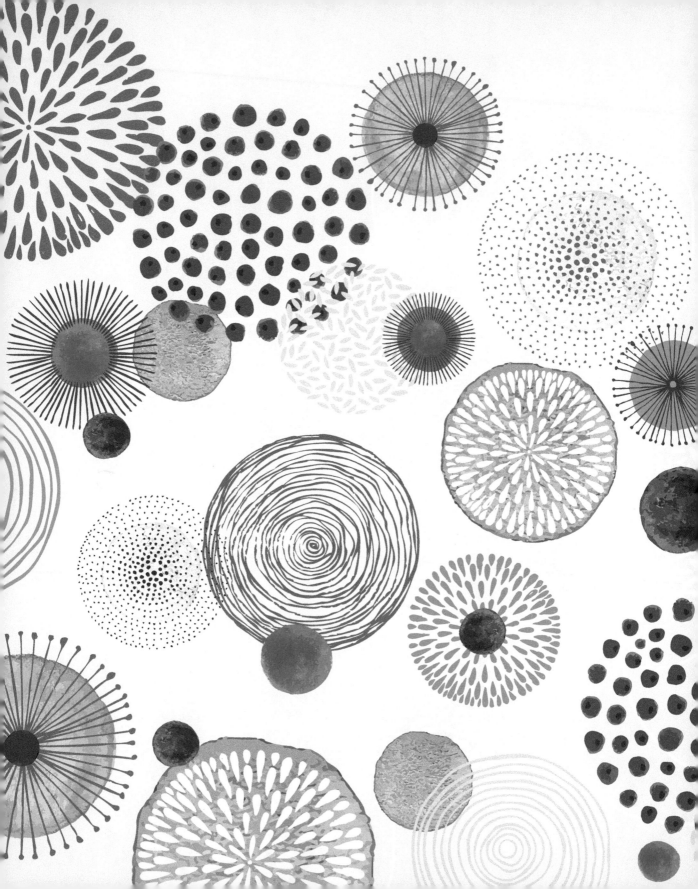

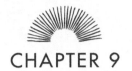

CHAPTER 9

Ankles, Feet, and Toes

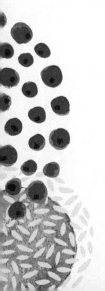

Vajrasana
(TOE STRETCH)

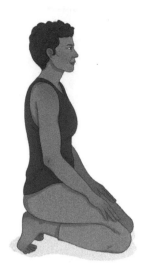

WARM-UP • PASSIVE

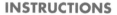

AFFECTED AREAS

Feet

Toes

GOOD FOR

✦ Stretching the soles of the feet

✦ Mobilizing the toes

INSTRUCTIONS

1. Start on all fours and tuck your toes with your feet parallel.
2. Sit back onto your heels with your toes tucked under.
3. Hold for five to 10 slow, deep breaths.

CHANGE IT UP

✦ Increase the intensity of the pose by letting your weight drop heavily onto your feet.

✦ Decrease the intensity of the pose by leaning forward or sitting up onto your knees.

✦ Add a tricep, shoulder, or wrist stretch to open the upper body.

REMEMBER

• Although this pose is not comfortable, it should not cause any sharp pain. If you feel any sharp pain, come out of the pose and, instead, stretch your feet by doing the Modified Virabhadrasana One (see page 84) at the wall or "Chair Toe Stand" (see page 82).

• If your feet feel very tight, consider rolling them out with a golf ball or tennis ball first.

Vrksasana

(TREE POSE)

ACTIVE
PROPS: OPTIONAL WALL

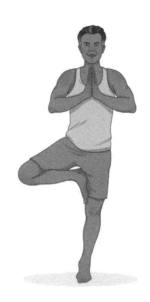

AFFECTED AREAS

Feet
Outer hips

GOOD FOR

✦ Balance
✦ Strengthening the outer hips

INSTRUCTIONS

1. Stand on your mat with your hands on your hips (or on the wall).
2. Bend your right knee and—keeping your hips squared forward—turn your right thigh out.
3. Lift your leg and place the sole of your right foot onto your ankle, calf, or upper thigh.
4. Hold for five to 10 slow, deep breaths.

CHANGE IT UP

✦ Increase the challenge by reaching your hands up the sky.
✦ Add support by placing your fingertips on the wall.
✦ If your balance feels steady, try closing your eyes.

REMEMBER

• Keeping your eyes focused on one point can help you balance.
• Wobbling in balancing poses is normal; it means your brain and nervous system are working.
• Press your lifted foot and opposite leg together strongly to create more support.

Garudasana
(EAGLE POSE)

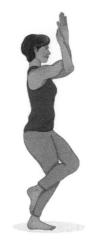
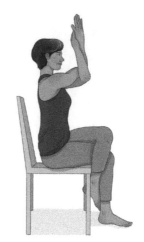

ACTIVE
PROPS: BLOCK; OPTIONAL WALL

AFFECTED AREAS

Adductors (strengthens)
Feet
Outer hips (strengthens)
Shoulders (stretches)

GOOD FOR

✦ Balance
✦ Strengthening the inner and outer hips

INSTRUCTIONS

1. Stand on your mat and reach your arms wide, parallel to the floor.
2. Exhale and cross your right arm under your left and hold on to opposite shoulders. (or leave the arms free and bring the fingertips to a wall).
3. Bend your left knee deeply and lift your right thigh over your left thigh. Bring your right toes onto a block (placed outside the left shin), or squeeze your thighs together and balance. If your foot and shin easily touch, then wrap your toes around your left calf.
4. Hold for five slow, deep breaths.

CHANGE IT UP

✦   If your elbows are stacked, then raise your forearms vertically and press the backs of your wrists together or wrap your forearms and press your palms together (see Garudasana Arms on page 32).

✦   Hinge forward to challenge your balance and come into a "nesting eagle."

✦   Give yourself more support by bringing your fingertips to the wall.

REMEMBER

•   Keeping your eyes focused on one point can help you balance.

•   If your torso is upright, relax your shoulders and draw your elbows forward to create a stretch between your shoulder blades.

Yogi Toe Massage

PASSIVE · COOLDOWN ·
PROPS: OPTIONAL BLOCK OR CHAIR

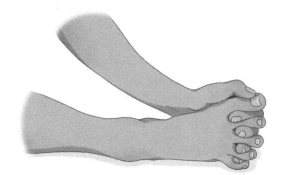

AFFECTED AREA

Feet

GOOD FOR

+ Stretching and strengthening the feet

INSTRUCTIONS

1. Sit cross-legged on your mat, block, or chair prop and draw one foot closer to you.
2. Interlace your fingers between your toes to stretch them apart. Roll your ankle in a circle five times. Repeat on the other side. (Note: If you are sitting in a chair, do the ankle rolls without using your hands.)
3. Let go of your toes and extend your legs long in front of you.
4. Slowly point and flex your feet 10 times.

CHANGE IT UP

+ Increase your support by doing this series seated in a chair.
+ Add intensity by interlacing your fingers between your toes up to the webbing of your feet.

REMEMBER

- The feet work hard! Treat them nicely, and they will become more pliable over time.
- Notice the position of your upper body while you're focusing on your feet, and keep your shoulders relaxed.

Viparita Karani
(LEGS-UP-THE-WALL POSE)

PASSIVE • COOLDOWN •
PROPS: WALL; OPTIONAL STRAP,
BOLSTER, PILLOW, OR CUSHION

AFFECTED AREAS

Circulatory System
Hamstrings (stretching)

GOOD FOR

+ Stretching the hamstrings
+ Activating a de-stress response
+ Lymphatic drainage and venous return (i.e., relieving swollen feet or calves)

INSTRUCTIONS

1. Lie on your side with your pelvis one to three feet away from the wall.
2. As you turn onto your back, move your legs up the wall.
3. Hold for five to 10 minutes.

CHANGE IT UP

+ Decrease the intensity of the hamstring stretch by moving your hips farther away from the wall or by placing a bolster or pillow beneath your hips.
+ Increase the hamstring stretch by bringing your hips closer to the wall (as long as they stay grounded).
+ For additional support, tie a strap or a scarf around your upper thighs or shins to let your hips relax.

REMEMBER

- Completely relax your body and let the floor support your weight.
- If your chin is lifting toward the sky, place a cushion beneath your head.

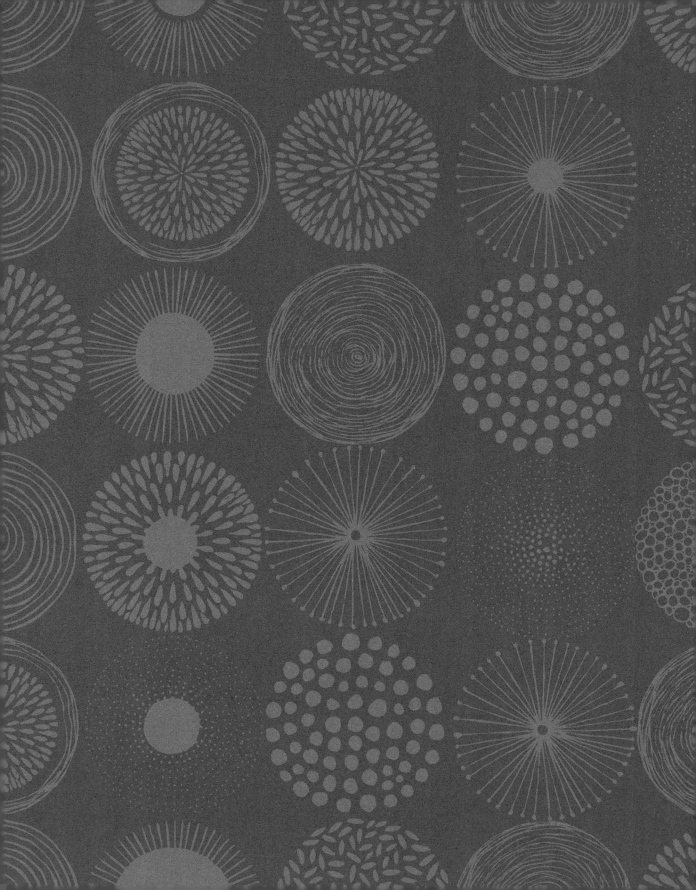

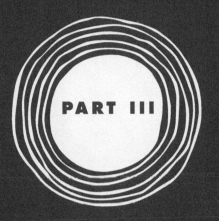

PART III

THE
SEQUENCES

In this section, we will put together the poses from the previous chapters into themed sequences to support your personal well-being. You can select a sequence based on your desired intention: providing support for your daily activities, addressing a particular area of your body, or targeting specific aches and pains. Each sequence will include an estimated time, describe the purpose of the sequence, list the poses, provide illustrations, and offer tips.

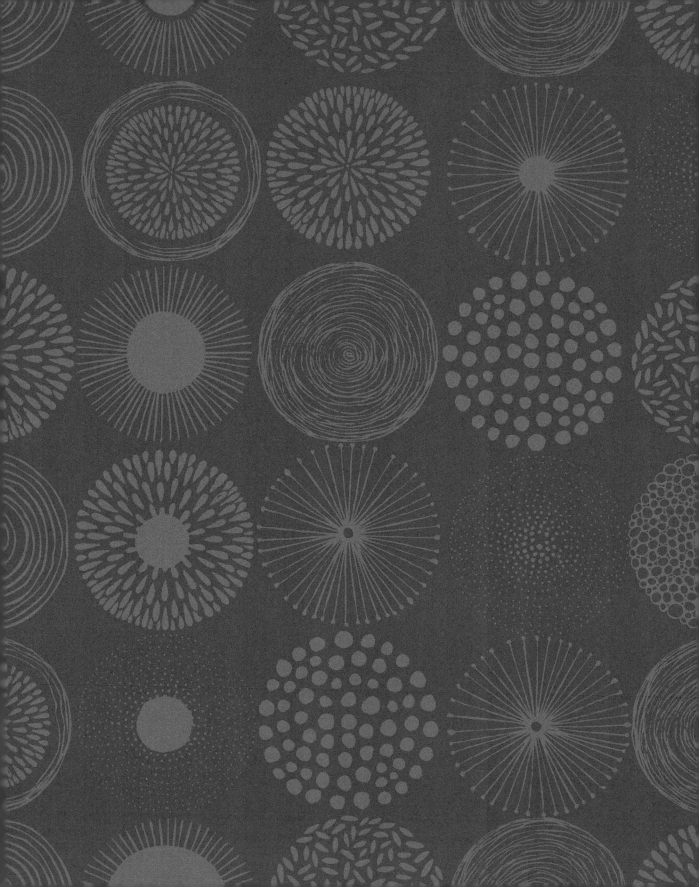

HOW TO USE THE SEQUENCES

Putting poses together into a sequence—rather than simply practicing one pose on its own—creates a cumulative beneficial effect. For example, by sequencing several shoulder stretches, you will move the shoulder in all directions rather than only one.

Linking poses together also gives you the opportunity to slow down, focus on your breath, and develop stability as you transition between postures. How you move *between* the poses is just as important as the pose itself. By slowing down and focusing on your transitions, you will develop more stability, balance, and awareness of your body. Remember, yoga isn't just about postures; it's about bringing mindfulness to each moment of your practice.

A Note on Breathing

Practicing yoga is a wonderful opportunity to remain conscious of your breath and cultivate mindfulness. Begin each sequence by first taking a few deep, centering breaths to become aware of your body and its sensations. As you move through your sequence, continue to breathe deeply and smoothly. Using your breath to stay present through each moment of your practice will help you de-stress, calm your mind, and nourish your mental health.

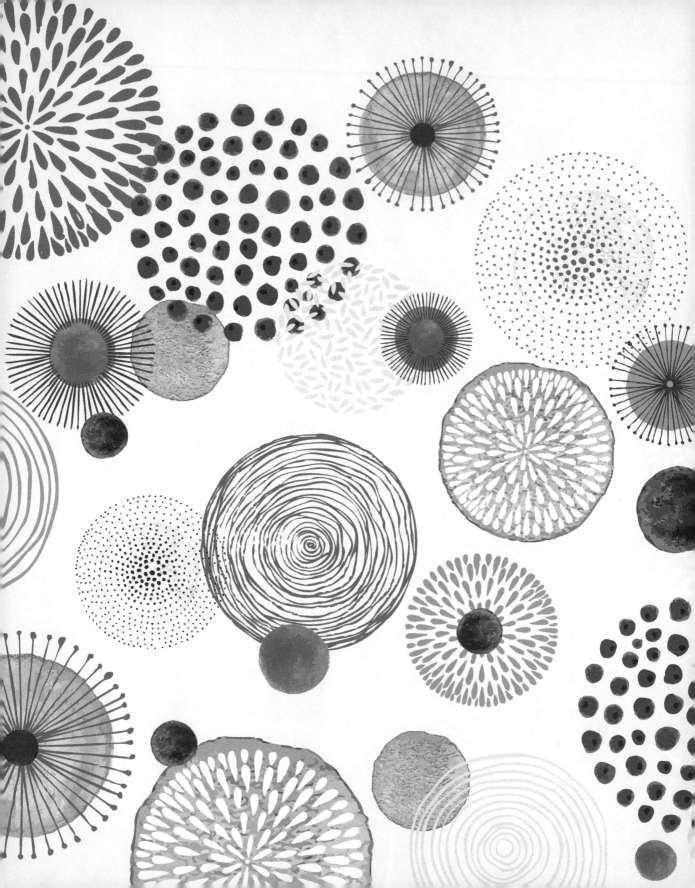

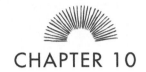

CHAPTER 10

Support for Everyday Activities

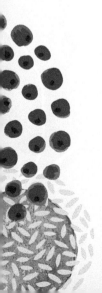

Yoga for Walking

TOTAL TIME: 20 MINUTES

GOOD FOR

Walking is excellent for improving leg strength and increasing your cardiovascular health, but it can often leave your hips and calves feeling tight. This sequence stretches out the areas of the body that are typically activated from walking.

REMEMBER Feel free to hold any stretch longer if it's feeling good. Take your time and breathe into each stretch fully.

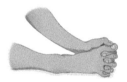

1

SUKHASANA
(see page 78):
five centering breaths.

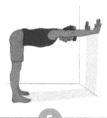

2

YOGI TOE MASSAGE
(see page 92):
about a minute per foot.

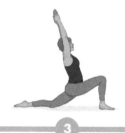

3

LOW LUNGE
(see page 70):
10 breaths on each
side. Repeat once.

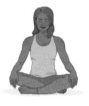

4

**MODIFIED
VIRABHADRASANA ONE**
(see page 84):
10 breaths on each side.

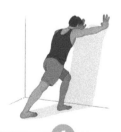

5

**SPINAL STRETCH
AT THE WALL**
(see page 40):
10 breaths.

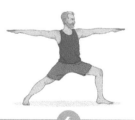

6

VIRABHADRASANA TWO
(see page 67):
10 breaths on each
side. Repeat once.

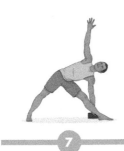

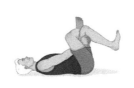

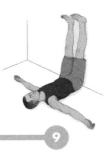

TRIKONASANA
(see page 69): 10 breaths
on each side. Repeat once.

THREAD THE NEEDLE
(see page 76):
10 breaths on each side.

VIPARITA KARANI
(see page 93): two
to five minutes.

Yoga for Sitting

TOTAL TIME: 35 MINUTES

GOOD FOR

Sitting can literally be a pain in the butt. We often sit for hours a day, whether we are working, driving, answering e-mails, or watching our favorite show. But too much sitting is hard on the legs, hips, and spine. This sequence is designed to bring some energy and vigor back into your lower body.

REMEMBER Take your time between postures to move carefully between each pose. Remember to bend deeply into your legs in the standing poses to build strength and encourage blood flow.

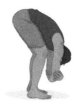

①

VIRASANA
(see page 83):
five centering breaths.

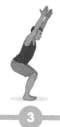

②

VAJRASANA
(see page 88):
Hold for 10 seconds, then
release and tap out the
tops of feet. Repeat once.

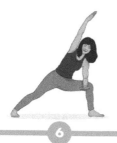

③

UTKATASANA
(see page 71):
10 breaths. Repeat twice.

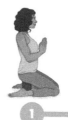

④

UTTANASANA
(see page 64):
10 breaths.

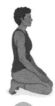

⑤

**UTKATASANA
WITH HEEL LIFT**
(see page 82):
10 seconds. Repeat once.

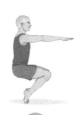

⑥

PARSVAKONASANA
(see page 68):
10 breaths on each
side. Repeat once.

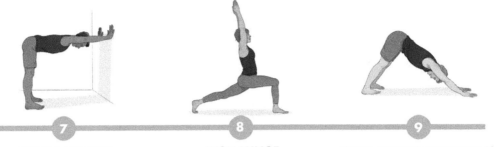

**SPINAL STRETCH
AT THE WALL**
(see page 40): 10 breaths.

HIGH LUNGE
(see page 70):
10 breaths on each side.

ADHO MUKHA SVANASANA
(see page 65): 10 breaths
(can substitute Cat/Cow Pose
[see page 50] if you wish).

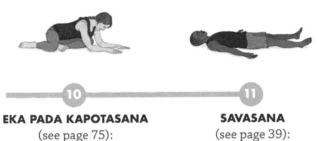

EKA PADA KAPOTASANA
(see page 75):
two minutes on each side.

SAVASANA
(see page 39):
five minutes.

Yoga for Gardening

TOTAL TIME: 35 MINUTES

GOOD FOR

Gardening is a wonderful and satisfying activity, but it often requires us to hunch over in a kneeling position for a long time as we manage the weeds. This sequence will help restore your body after time in your garden.

> **REMEMBER** Gardening encourages us to hunch over, so use each pose as an opportunity to find space and breath, particularly in the front of your body and chest.

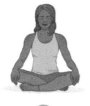

SUKHASANA
(see page 78):
five centering breaths.

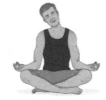

SIMPLE NECK STRETCHES
(see page 30):
five breaths for each stretch.

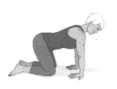

WRIST STRETCH
(see page 60):
10 breaths.

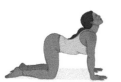 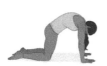

CAT/COW POSE
(see page 50):
10 rounds. Inhale for
Cow, exhale for Cat.

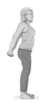

YOGA MUDRA
(see page 33): Hold for one
minute with each inter-
lock of your fingers.

**SPINAL STRETCH
AT THE WALL**
(see page 40): Hold
for 10 breaths.

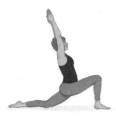

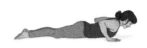

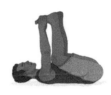

7

LOW OR HIGH LUNGE
(see page 70): Hold for 10 breaths on each side.

8

PRASARITA PADOTTANASANA
(see page 72): Hold for 10 breaths.

9

BHUJANGASANA
(see page 42): Hold for five breaths. Repeat twice.

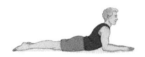

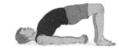

10

SPHINX POSE
(see page 46): Hold for five breaths.

11

SETU BANDHA SARVANGASANA
(see page 51): Hold for five breaths. Repeat twice.

12

ANANDA BALASANA
(see page 77): Hold for 10 breaths.

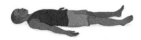

13

SAVASANA
(see page 39): five minutes.

Yoga for Lifting Heavy Things

TOTAL TIME: 20 MINUTES

GOOD FOR

Lifting heavy objects properly requires allowing the hips, knees, and ankles to flex so that the spine can remain straight and well aligned. This sequence is designed to increase awareness and mobility in these joints so that they can move freely.

REMEMBER As you move through this sequence, focus on hinging from your hips and finding length through your whole spine.

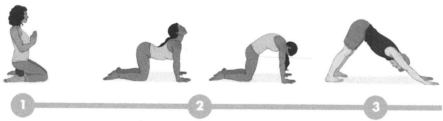

VIRASANA (see page 83) or
SUKHASANA (see page 78):
five centering breaths.

CAT/COW POSE
(see page 50): 10 rounds.
Inhale for Cow, exhale for Cat.

ADHO MUKHA SVANASANA
(see page 65): five breaths.
Bend one knee and press
through the opposite foot to
stretch the back of the calf.

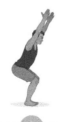

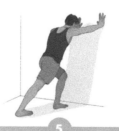

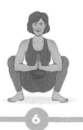

UTKATASANA (see page 71):
Inhale to stand in Tadasana
(see page 38), then exhale
to sit back into chair.
Repeat five times.

**MODIFIED
VIRABHADRASANA ONE**
(see page 84):
10 breaths on each side.

MALASANA
(see page 85):
10 breaths.

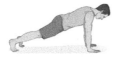 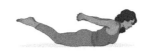 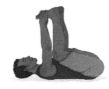

7　　　　　　　　　**8**　　　　　　　　　**9**

PHALAKASANA
(see page 58):
five to 10 breaths.

SALABHASANA
(see page 44):
five breaths. Repeat twice.

ANANDA BALASANA
(see page 77):
10 breaths.

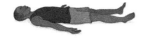

10

SAVASANA
(see page 39):
five minutes.

Yoga for Shoveling Snow

TOTAL TIME: 20 MINUTES

GOOD FOR

Shoveling snow is great exercise, but it can leave you feeling tight through the shoulders and spine from unilateral twisting. This sequence will balance you out.

REMEMBER Use your inhale to find more space in each posture and make sure to exhale completely. Be sure to breathe deeply and use the breath to support you during twists.

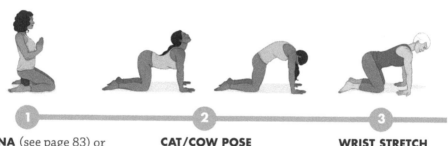

VIRASANA (see page 83) or **SUKHASANA** (see page 78): five centering breaths.

CAT/COW POSE (see page 50): 10 rounds. Inhale for Cow, exhale for Cat.

WRIST STRETCH (see page 60): 10 breaths.

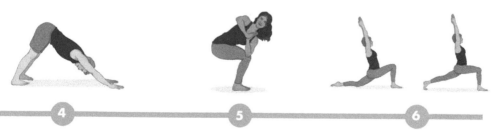

ADHO MUKHA SVANASANA (see page 65): 10 breaths.

PARIVRTTA UTKATASANA (see page 55): five breaths on each side. Inhale to lengthen and exhale to twist.

LOW OR HIGH LUNGE (see page 70): Hold for 10 breaths on each side.

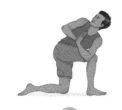

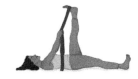

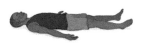

7

**PARIVRTTA
PARSVAKONASANA**
(see page 54): five breaths
on each side. Inhale to
lengthen and exhale to twist.

8

**SUPTA HASTA
PADANGUSTHASANA SERIES**
(see page 73): Hold each
stretch for five to 10 breaths.

9

SAVASANA
(see page 39):
five minutes.

Yoga for Yard Work

TOTAL TIME: 15 MINUTES

GOOD FOR

Raking leaves, trimming trees, or landscaping can be a great full-body workout. However, this kind of physical exercise can leave both your shoulders and hips tight. This post-yard-work sequence is designed to help you stretch out those tight spots.

REMEMBER In this sequence, focus on keeping your chest spacious and open.

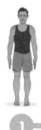

1

TADASANA
(see page 38):
five centering breaths.

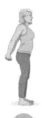

2

YOGA MUDRA
(see page 33): five breaths,
then change inter-
lock of fingers and take
five more breaths.

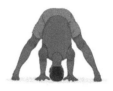

3

**PRASARITA
PADOTTANASANA**
(see page 72):
10 breaths.

4

LOW OR HIGH LUNGE
(see page 70):
10 breaths on each side.

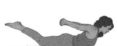

5

SALABHASANA
(see page 44): five
breaths. Repeat twice.

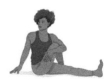

6

ARDHA MATSYENDRASANA
(see page 52): five breaths
on each side. Inhale to
lengthen, exhale to twist.

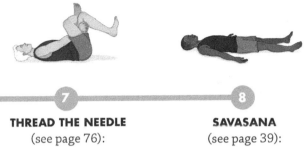

THREAD THE NEEDLE
(see page 76):
10 breaths on each side.

SAVASANA
(see page 39):
five minutes.

Yoga for Needlepoint, Reading, Knitting, or Crafts

TOTAL TIME: 40 MINUTES

GOOD FOR

This active sequence is a lovely antidote for when you do work with your hands while sitting, such as needlepoint, reading, knitting, or crafts.

REMEMBER This sequence has several transitions. Stay present and rooted through your feet as you move between the postures. Feel free to keep your hands on the floor or on a chair for support.

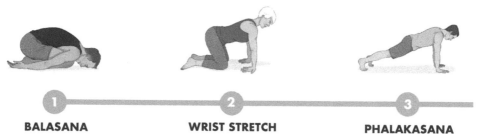

1

BALASANA
(see page 41):
five centering breaths.

2

WRIST STRETCH
(see page 60):
10 breaths.

3

PHALAKASANA
(see page 58):
five to 10 breaths.

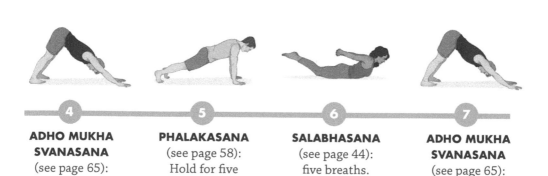

4

**ADHO MUKHA
SVANASANA**
(see page 65):
10 breaths

5

PHALAKASANA
(see page 58):
Hold for five
breaths, then lower
to the floor.

6

SALABHASANA
(see page 44):
five breaths.
Repeat twice.

7

**ADHO MUKHA
SVANASANA**
(see page 65):
Hold for five
slow breaths.

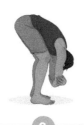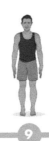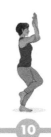

8	**9**	**10**
UTTANASANA	**TADASANA**	**GARUDASANA**
(see page 64): Walk your feet forward to your hands to Uttanasana. Hold for five breaths.	(see page 38): Slowly rise up to stand in Tadasana. Hold for three to five breaths.	(see page 90): five breaths on each side.

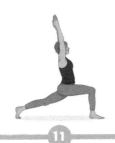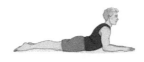

11	**12**	**13**
HIGH LUNGE	**SPHINX POSE**	**USTRASANA**
(see page 70): Lower hands to the floor, stepping back into High Lunge. Take five breaths. Repeat on the other side.	(see page 46): five breaths.	(see page 48): three breaths. Repeat once (or repeat Sphinx Pose).

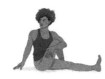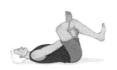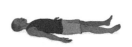

14	**15**	**16**	**17**
ARDHA MATSYENDRASANA	**THREAD THE NEEDLE**	**ANANDA BALASANA**	**SAVASANA**
(see page 52): 10 breaths on each side.	(see page 76): 10 breaths on each side.	(see page 77): 10 breaths.	(see page 39): five minutes.

Yoga for Playing Cards or Games

TOTAL TIME: 25 MINUTES

GOOD FOR

This sequence helps release shoulder and neck tension from playing cards or games. It also helps get some energy back into your legs after sitting for any period of time.

REMEMBER When doing neck or arm stretches, it can be tempting to drop your head forward or hunch the back. Make sure to keep your chest open and lifted. When you do arm stretches, keep your head aligned with your spine.

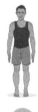

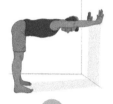

TADASANA
(see page 38):
five centering breaths.

SIMPLE NECK STRETCHES (STANDING OR SITTING)
(see page 30): five breaths for each stretch.

SPINAL STRETCH AT THE WALL
(see page 40):
10 breaths.

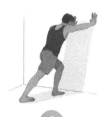
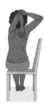
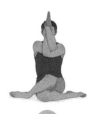

MODIFIED VIRABHADRASANA ONE AT THE WALL
(see page 84): five breaths on each side.

GOMUKHASANA ARMS (SITTING OR STANDING)
(see page 31): five breaths on each side.

GARUDASANA ARMS (SITTING OR STANDING)
(see page 32): five breaths on each side.

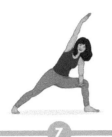

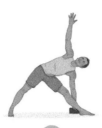

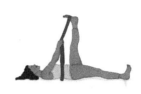

7

8

9

PARSVAKONASANA
(see page 68): five breaths
on each side. Repeat once.

TRIKONASANA
(see page 69): five
breaths on each side.

**SUPTA HASTA
PADANGUSTHASANA SERIES**
(see page 73): five breaths
(or more if desired)
in each stretch.

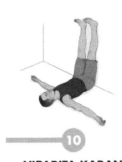

10

VIPARITA KARANI
(see page 93) or Savasana
(see page 39): five min-
utes. Choose the pose
that feels good.

Yoga for Waking Up

TOTAL TIME: 20 TO 30 MINUTES

GOOD FOR

This flowing sequence helps you wake your body up to prepare for your day.

REMEMBER During this flow-style sequence, focus on moving with your breath. Take your time and add breaths as needed to move smoothly between the postures. Decrease the intensity of the sequence by holding the postures for a shorter length of time; increase the intensity of the sequence by holding the postures longer. Feel free to use support (chair or wall) for the transitions.

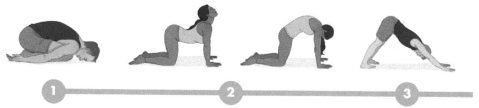

BALASANA
(see page 41):
five centering breaths.

CAT/COW POSE
(see page 50): 10 rounds.
Inhale for Cow, exhale for Cat.

ADHO MUKHA SVANASANA
(see page 65): 10 breaths
(can substitute Cat/
Cow Pose if you wish).

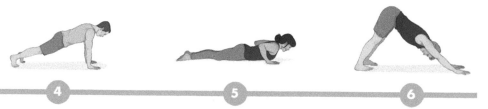

PHALAKASANA
(see page 58): Hold for
five breaths, then exhale
and lower to the floor.

BHUJANGASANA
(see page 42): Inhale for one
breath, exhale to lower down.

ADHO MUKHA SVANASANA
(see page 65): 10 breaths
(can substitute Cat/
Cow Pose if you wish).

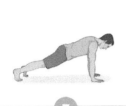
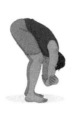
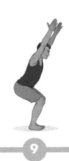

7

Repeat steps 4 to 6 three times.

8

WALK FORWARD TO UTTANASANA (see page 64): five breaths.

9

UTKATASANA (see page 71): five breaths. Repeat twice.

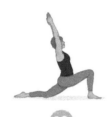
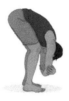
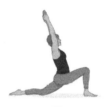

10

STEP ONE FOOT BACK INTO LOW LUNGE (see page 70): five breaths.

11

Step forward to **UTTANASANA**: five breaths.

12

Step the opposite foot back to **LOW LUNGE**: five breaths.

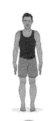
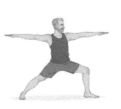
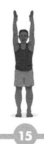
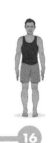

13

Step forward to **UTTANASANA**, then stand into **TADASANA** (see page 38).

14

VIRABHADRASANA TWO (see page 67): five breaths on each side. Repeat once.

15

TADASANA Inhale and reach up (see page 34). Lower into Tadasana; five times.

16

TADASANA five deep centering breaths.

Yoga for Bedtime

TOTAL TIME: 25 MINUTES

GOOD FOR

This nourishing and calming sequence is designed to help your body prepare for a good night's rest.

REMEMBER Allow the floor to support your body weight. Use each pose as an opportunity to sink into your breath and relax more deeply.

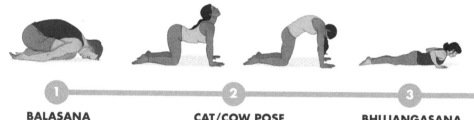

BALASANA
(see page 41):
five deep breaths.

CAT/COW POSE
(see page 50): 10 rounds.
Inhale for Cow, exhale for Cat.

BHUJANGASANA
(see page 42): three
breaths. Repeat twice.

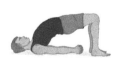
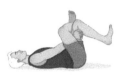
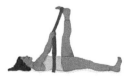

**SETU BANDHA
SARVANGASANA**
(see page 51): Lift your hips as
you inhale, exhale as you roll
down. Repeat three times.

THREAD THE NEEDLE
(see page 76):
10 breaths on each side.

**SUPTA HASTA
PADANGUSTHASANA SERIES**
(see page 73): Hold each
stretch for five to 10 breaths.

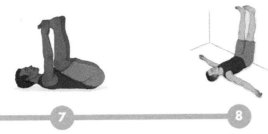

ANANDA BALASANA
(see page 77): Hold
for 10 breaths.

VIPARITA KARANI
(see page 93) or Savasana
(see page 39): five minutes.

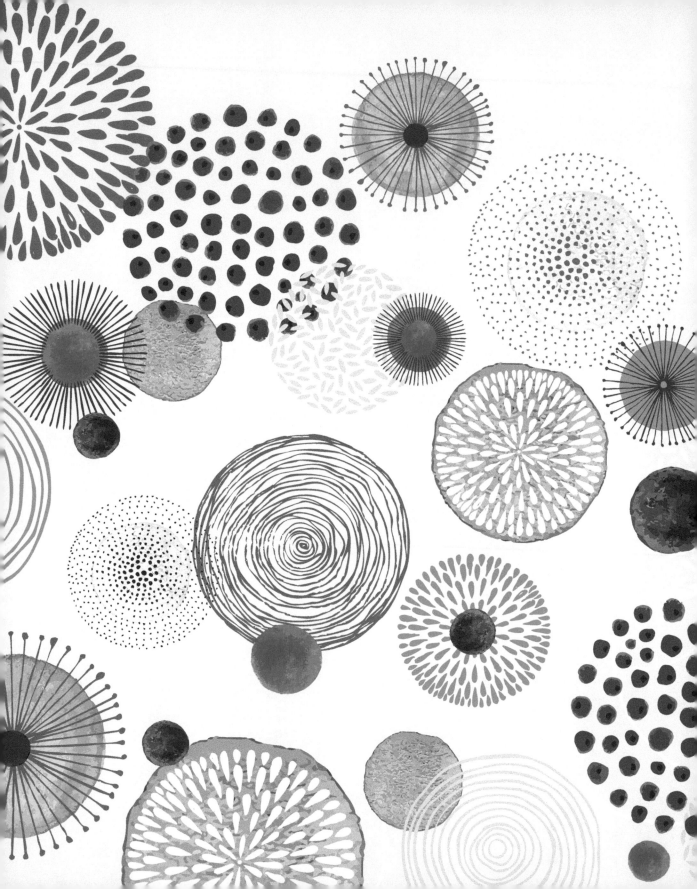

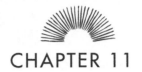

Active Living

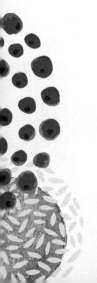

Yoga for Running

TOTAL TIME: 40 MINUTES

GOOD FOR

Running is excellent for improving leg strength and increasing your cardiovascular health, but it can often leave your hips and legs tight. This sequence stretches out the areas of your body that are typically left feeling tight from jogging and running.

REMEMBER Take your time and lengthen your breath to actively release your muscles.

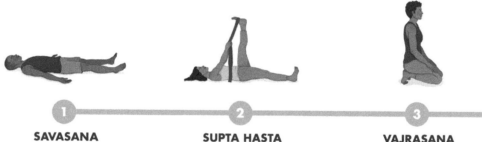

1

SAVASANA
(see page 39):
five centering breaths.

2

SUPTA HASTA
PADANGUSTHASANA SERIES
(see page 73): Hold each
stretch for five to 10 breaths.

3

VAJRASANA
(see page 88): Hold for 10 seconds, then release and tap out
the tops of feet. Repeat once.

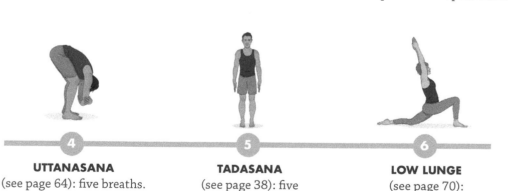

4

UTTANASANA
(see page 64): five breaths.

5

TADASANA
(see page 38): five
deep breaths.

6

LOW LUNGE
(see page 70):
10 breaths on each side.

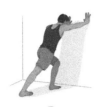

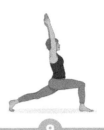

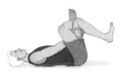

7

MODIFIED VIRABHADRASANA ONE
(see page 84):
five breaths on each side.

8

SPINAL STRETCH AT THE WALL
(see page 40): Hold
for 10 breaths.

9

HIGH LUNGE
(see page 70): five
breaths on each side.

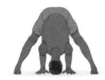

10

PRASARITA PADOTTANASANA
(see page 72): 10 breaths.

11

MALASANA
(see page 85):
five breaths.

12

THREAD THE NEEDLE
(see page 76): five
breaths on each side.

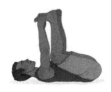

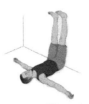

13

ANANDA BALASANA
(see page 77):
10 breaths.

14

VIPARITA KARANI
(see page 93):
five minutes.

Yoga for Swimming

TOTAL TIME: 20 MINUTES

GOOD FOR

Swimming is an excellent, low-impact activity for strengthening your cardiovascular health. This sequence stretches out the areas of your body—shoulder, neck, and hamstrings—that are typically left feeling tight from swimming.

> **REMEMBER** When doing shoulder stretches, it can become tempting to arch your upper back or drop your head forward. Keep your chest lifted and your head aligned with your spine.

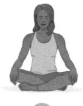 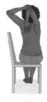

1

SUKHASANA
(see page 78): Add an Uttanasana (see page 64); hold for 5 breaths. Re-cross legs and repeat.

2

SIMPLE NECK STRETCHES
(see page 30): Stay in Sukhasana. Hold each stretch for five breaths.

3

GOMUKHASANA ARMS
(see page 31): Stay in Sukhasana. Hold for five breaths on each side.

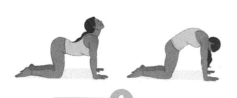 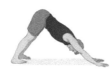

4

CAT/COW POSE
(see page 50): 10 rounds. Inhale for Cow, exhale for Cat.

5

ADHO MUKHA SVANASANA
(see page 65): 10 breaths (can substitute Cat/Cow Pose if you wish).

6

UTTANASANA
(see page 64): five breaths.

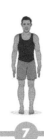

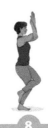

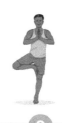

7

YOGA MUDRA

(see page 33): five breaths with each inter-lock of your fingers.

8

GARUDASANA

(see page 90): five breaths on each side.

9

VRKSASANA

(see page 89): five breaths on each side.

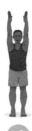

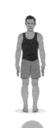

10

URDHVA HASTASANA

(see page 34): Inhale and reach arms up to Urdhva Hastasana. As you exhale, lower your arms to Tadasana. Repeat five times.

11

TADASANA

five centering breaths.

Yoga for Biking: Long

TOTAL TIME: 50 MINUTES

GOOD FOR

Biking is excellent for improving leg strength and increasing your cardiovascular health, though it might leave you feeling hunched over and tight in the glutes and hamstrings. This sequence targets the hips and spine to balance out your body from cycling.

REMEMBER This series involves several transitions. Take your time to mindfully move between the shapes.

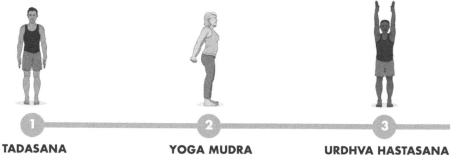

TADASANA
(see page 38):
five centering breaths.

YOGA MUDRA
(see page 33): Hold for five breaths with each inter-lock of your fingers.

URDHVA HASTASANA
(see page 34): Inhale
to lift your arms.

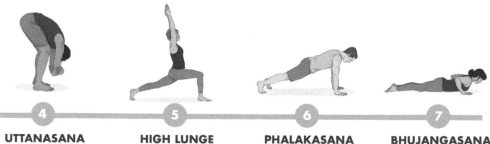

UTTANASANA
(see page 64): Exhale
to Uttanasana. Hold
for five breaths.

HIGH LUNGE
(see page 70): five
breaths on each side.

PHALAKASANA
(see page 58): Hold
for five to 10 breaths.

BHUJANGASANA
(see page 42): three
breaths. Repeat twice.

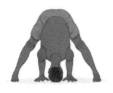

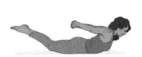

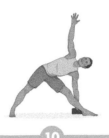

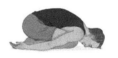

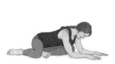

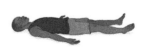

8

SALABHASANA
(see page 44): three
breaths. Repeat twice.

9

**ADHO MUKHA
SVANASANA**
(see page 65): Hold
for 10 breaths.

10

TRIKONASANA
(see page 69): Hold for
five breaths on each
side. Repeat once.

11

**PRASARITA
PADOTTANASANA**
(see page 72): Hold
for 10 breaths.

12

**PARIVRTTA
PARSVAKONASANA**
(see page 54):
Pause on each side.
Inhale to lengthen;
exhale to twist.

13

USTRASANA
(see page 48): three
breaths. Repeat twice.

14

BALASANA
(see page 41):
five breaths.

15

**EKA PADA
KAPOTASANA**
(see page 75):
10 breaths on
each side.

16

**SUPTA HASTA
PADANGUSTHASANA
SERIES** (see page 73):
Hold each stretch for
five to 10 breaths.

17

**ANANDA
BALASANA**
(see page 77):
10 breaths.

18

SAVASANA
(see page 39):
five minutes.

Yoga for Biking: Short

TOTAL TIME: 15 MINUTES

GOOD FOR

This modified version of the 50-minute series (see page 126) is a great quick fix for stretching out the muscles that get tight through cycling, such as the glutes, hamstrings, and calves.

REMEMBER Although this series is shorter, take your time with each stretch. Feel free to hold the poses longer for particularly tight spots.

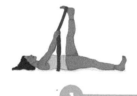
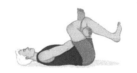
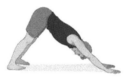

1

2

3

SUPTA HASTA PADANGUSTHASANA SERIES (see page 73): Hold each stretch for five to 10 breaths.

THREAD THE NEEDLE (see page 76): 10 breaths on each side.

ADHO MUKHA SVANASANA (see page 65): Hold for 10 breaths. Pedal your feet to stretch your calves.

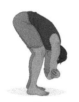
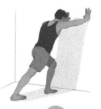
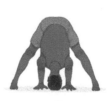
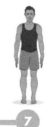

4

5

6

7

UTTANASANA (see page 64): 10 breaths.

MODIFIED VIRABHADRASANA ONE (see page 84): Hold for five breaths on each side.

PRASARITA PADOTTANASANA (see page 72): 10 breaths.

TADASANA (see page 38): five centering breaths.

Yoga for Golf

GOOD FOR

Golfing is excellent for hand-eye coordination and full-body conditioning, but its unilateral movements can leave you feeling tight through the spine, neck, and shoulders. This series is designed to help you improve and recover from your golf game by improving your core, balance, and spinal rotation.

REMEMBER When twisting, make sure your pelvis, spine, and head remain aligned. Inhale to create space and lengthen your spine, then exhale to twist.

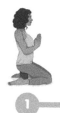
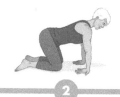
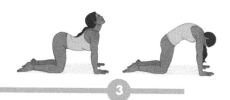

1

VIRASANA
(see page 83) or
Sukhasana (see page 78):
five centering breaths.

2

WRIST STRETCH
(see page 60): Hold
for five breaths.

3

CAT/COW POSE
(see page 50):
10 rounds. Inhale for
Cow, exhale for Cat.

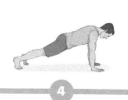
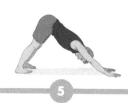
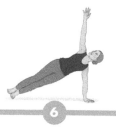

4

PHALAKASANA
(see page 58):
Hold for five to 10
breaths. Repeat twice.

5

**ADHO MUKHA
SVANASANA**
(see page 65): 10 breaths
(can substitute Cat/
Cow Pose if you wish).

6

VASISTHASANA
(see page 59): five
breaths on each side.

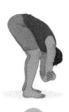
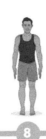
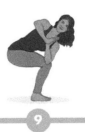

7

UTTANASANA
(see page 64):
10 breaths.

8

TADASANA
(see page 38) with Simple
Neck Stretches (see page 30):
five breaths for each stretch.

9

PARIVRTTA UTKATASANA
(see page 55):
five breaths on each
side. Inhale to lengthen
and exhale to twist.

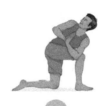
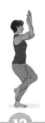

10

LOW OR HIGH LUNGE
(see page 70):
five breaths on each side.

11

**PARIVRTTA
PARSVAKONASANA**
(see page 54): five breaths
on each side. Inhale to
lengthen and exhale to twist.

12

GARUDASANA
(see page 90): five
breaths on each side.

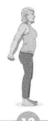
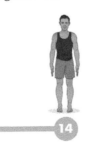

13

YOGA MUDRA
(see page 33):
five breaths with each
interlock of your fingers.

14

TADASANA
(see page 38):
five centering breaths.

Yoga for Tennis

TOTAL TIME: 25 MINUTES

GOOD FOR

This recovery sequence targets the muscles that get tight from playing tennis, such as the hamstrings, glutes, and chest.

REMEMBER When stretching out your hamstrings, be careful to not lock your knee. Instead, keep a microbend in your knee to engage your quadriceps.

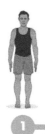

1

TADASANA
(see page 38):
five centering breaths.

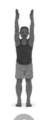

2

YOGA MUDRA
(see page 33):
five breaths with each interlock of the fingers.

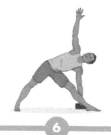

3

URDHVA HASTASANA
(see page 34):
five breaths.

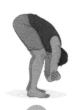

4

UTTANASANA
(see page 64):
10 breaths.

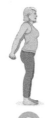

5

VIRABHADRASANA TWO
(see page 67):
five breaths on each side.

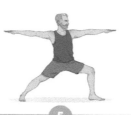

6

TRIKONASANA
(see page 69):
five breaths on each side.

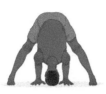

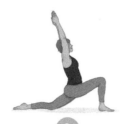

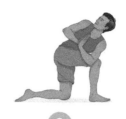

7
**PRASARITA
PADOTTANASANA**
(see page 72):
10 breaths.

8
LOW LUNGE
(see page 70):
five breaths on each side.

9
**PARIVRTTA
PARSVAKONASANA**
(see page 54):
five breaths on each
side. Inhale to lengthen
and exhale to twist.

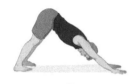

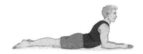

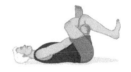

10
ADHO MUKHA SVANASANA
(see page 65): 10 breaths
(can substitute Cat/Cow Pose
[see page 50] if you wish).

11
SPHINX POSE
(see page 46):
five breaths. Repeat once.

12
THREAD THE NEEDLE
(see page 76):
10 breaths on each side.

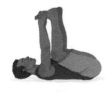

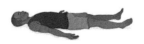

13
ANANDA BALASANA
(see page 77):
10 breaths.

14
SAVASANA
(see page 39):
five minutes.

Yoga for Softball or Baseball

TOTAL TIME: 30 MINUTES

GOOD FOR

Softball and baseball can be excellent for cardiovascular health and whole-body conditioning. This series is designed to help you improve and recover from your game by targeting your core, balance, and spinal mobility.

REMEMBER When transitioning from the floor to standing or vice versa, hinge from your hips and use the strength of your legs.

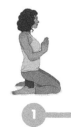
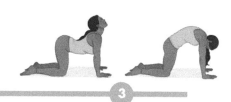

1

VIRASANA
(see page 83) or
Sukhasana (see page 78):
five centering breaths.

2

WRIST STRETCH
(see page 60):
five breaths.

3

CAT/COW POSE
(see page 50):
10 rounds. Inhale for
Cow, exhale for Cat.

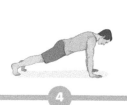
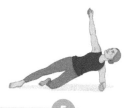
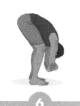

4

PHALAKASANA
(see page 58):
five to 10 breaths.

5

VASISTHASANA
(see page 59): five to
10 breaths on each side.

6

UTTANASANA
(see page 64):
10 breaths.

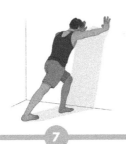

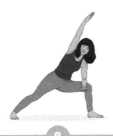

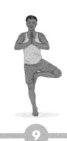

7

MODIFIED VIRABHADRASANA ONE
(see page 84):
10 breaths on each side.

8

PARSVAKONASANA
(see page 68):
five breaths on each side.

9

VRKSASANA
(see page 89):
five breaths on each side.

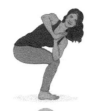

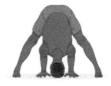

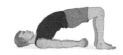

10

PARIVRTTA UTKATASANA
(see page 55): five breaths
on each side. Inhale to
lengthen and exhale to twist.

11

PRASARITA PADOTTANASANA
(see page 72):
10 breaths.

12

SETU BANDHA SARVANGASANA
(see page 51): five
breaths. Repeat twice.

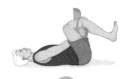

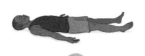

13

THREAD THE NEEDLE
(see page 76):
10 breaths on each side.

14

SAVASANA
(see page 39):
five minutes.

Yoga for Dancing

TOTAL TIME: 30 MINUTES

GOOD FOR

Like yoga, dancing encourages both strength and flexibility and improves your coordination. This sequence will support your dance moves by targeting your hamstrings and balance.

REMEMBER When stretching your hamstrings, it can be easy to lock your knee and disengage your quadriceps. Keep a soft bend to the back of your knee and engage your thigh muscles.

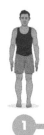

1

TADASANA
(see page 38):
five centering breaths.

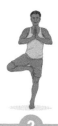

2

VRKSASANA
(see page 89):
five breaths on each side.

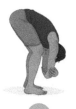

3

UTTANASANA
(see page 64):
10 breaths.

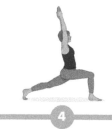

4

HIGH LUNGE
(see page 70):
five breaths on each side.

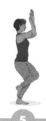

5

GARUDASANA
(see page 90):
five breaths on each side.

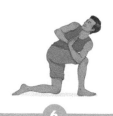

6

**PARIVRTTA
PARSVAKONASANA**
(see page 54): five breaths
on each side. Inhale to
lengthen and exhale to twist.

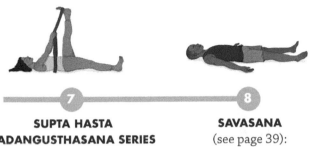

**SUPTA HASTA
PADANGUSTHASANA SERIES**
(see page 73): Hold each
stretch for five to 10 breaths.

SAVASANA
(see page 39):
five minutes.

Yoga for Skiing

TOTAL TIME: 30 MINUTES

GOOD FOR

Skiing is a wonderful sport for experiencing the outdoors and strengthening your legs. This sequence will help build your leg muscles for ski season.

REMEMBER This sequence deliberately includes long holds to build strength and resilience in your legs. When you become uncomfortable, focus on your breath and see if you can stay in the posture for another one or two breaths. To ramp up the fire, keep your knee bent in the transition between Virabhadrasana Two and Parsvakonasana.

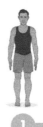

TADASANA
(see page 38):
five centering breaths.

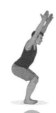

UTKATASANA
(see page 71):
five breaths. Repeat
four times.

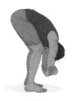

UTTANASANA
(see page 64):
10 breaths.

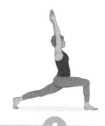

HIGH LUNGE
(see page 70):
five breaths on each side.

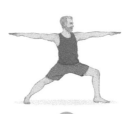

VIRABHADRASANA TWO
(see page 67):
five breaths on each
side. Repeat once.

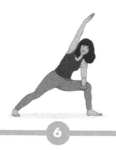

PARSVAKONASANA
(see page 68):
five breaths on each
side. Repeat once.

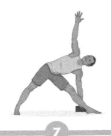

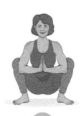

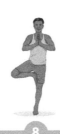

7

TRIKONASANA
(see page 69):
five breaths on each
side. Repeat once.

8

VRKSASANA
(see page 89):
five breaths on each side.

9

MALASANA
(see page 85):
10 breaths.

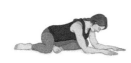

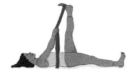

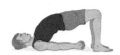

10

EKA PADA KAPOTASANA
(see page 75) or Thread
the Needle (see page 76):
10 breaths on each side.

11

**SUPTA HASTA
PADANGUSTHASANA**
(see page 73): Hold each
stretch for five to 10 breaths.

12

**SETU BANDHA
SARVANGASANA**
(see page 51): Hold for five
breaths. Repeat twice.

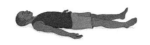

13

SAVASANA
(see page 39):
five minutes.

Yoga for General Exercise Recovery

TOTAL TIME: 60 MINUTES

GOOD FOR

This delicious, full-body sequence is a nourishing practice to stretch and strengthen your entire body.

REMEMBER This series involves several transitions. Take your time to mindfully move between each pose.

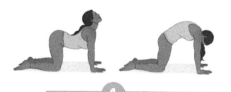

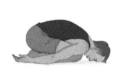

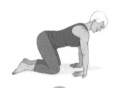

BALASANA
(see page 41):
10 centering breaths.

VAJRASANA
(see page 88): five breaths,
then tap out the tops of
your feet. Repeat once.

WRIST STRETCH
(see page 60):
five breaths.

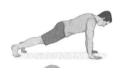

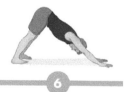

CAT/COW POSE
(see page 50):
10 rounds. Inhale for
Cow, exhale for Cat.

PHALAKASANA
(see page 58):
five to 10 breaths.

ADHO MUKHA SVANASANA
(see page 65):
five breaths.

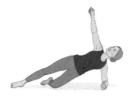
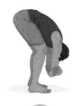

7

VASISTHASANA
(see page 59):
five to 10 breaths.

8

ADHO MUKHA SVANASANA
five breaths.

9

UTTANASANA
(see page 64):
five breaths.

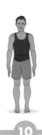
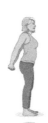
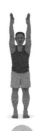

10

TADASANA
(see page 38):
one breath.

11

YOGA MUDRA
(see page 33):
five breaths with each
interlock of the hands.

12

URDHVA HASTASANA
(see page 34):
one breath.

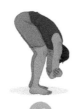
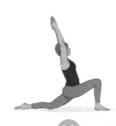

13

UTTANASANA
one breath.

14

LOW LUNGE
(see page 70): five breaths
on each side. Step forward to
Uttanasana between sides.

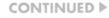

CONTINUED ▶

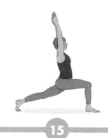

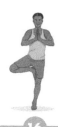

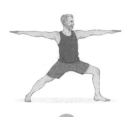

15

HIGH LUNGE

five breaths on each side.
Step forward to Uttana-
sana between sides.

16

VRKSASANA

(see page 89):
five breaths on each
side. Repeat once.

17

VIRABHADRASANA TWO

(see page 67):
five breaths on each
side. Repeat once.

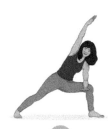

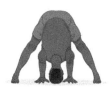

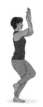

18

PARSVAKONASANA

(see page 68):
five breaths.

19

**PRASARITA
PADOTTANASANA**

(see page 72):
10 breaths.

20

GARUDASANA

(see page 90):
five breaths on each side.

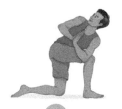

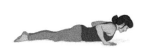

21

PARIVRTTA UTKATASANA

(see page 55): five breaths
on each side. Inhale to
lengthen and exhale to twist.

22

**PARIVRTTA
PARSVAKONASANA**

(see page 54): five breaths
on each side. Inhale to
lengthen and exhale to twist.

23

BHUJANGASANA

(see page 42):
three breaths.
Repeat twice.

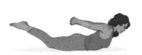

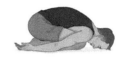

24

25

26

SALABHASANA
(see page 44):
three breaths.
Repeat twice.

USTRASANA
(see page 48):
three breaths.
Repeat twice.

BALASANA
10 breaths.

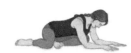

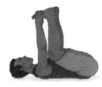

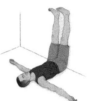

27

28

29

EKA PADA KAPOTASANA
(see page 75) or Thread
the Needle (see page 76):
10 breaths on each side.

ANANDA BALASANA
(see page 77):
10 breaths.

VIPARITA KARANI
(see page 93):
10 breaths.

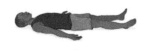

30

SAVASANA
(see page 39):
five minutes.

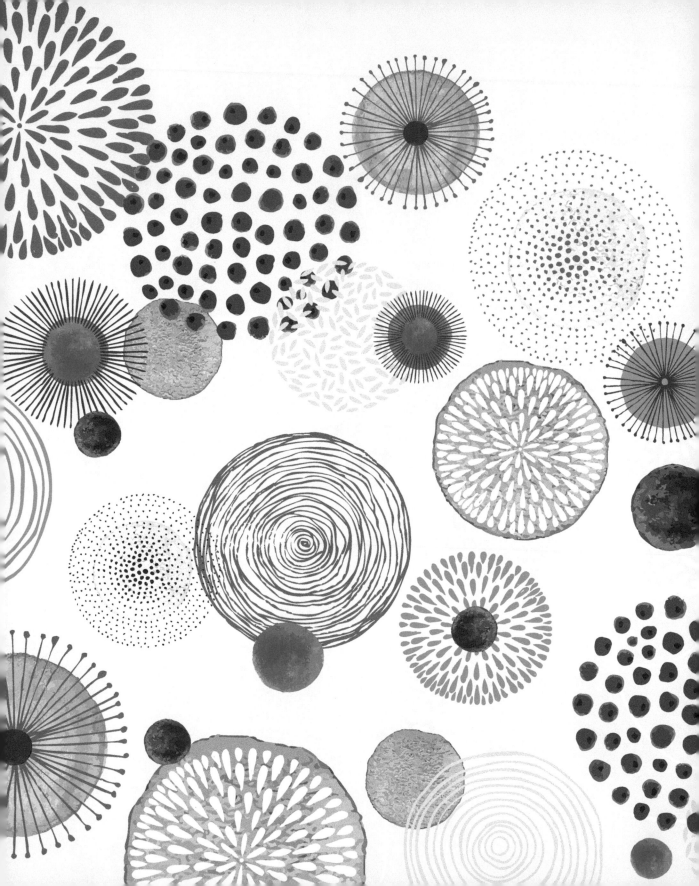

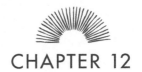

CHAPTER 12

Injury Recovery

A note on all injury recovery sequences: These sequences are intended to use yoga activities to sensibly support a practitioner who is generally healthy and working with a chronic issue. These sequences are not meant to replace therapeutic exercise, address acute conditions, or be construed as medical advice. Always follow your doctor's recommendations and modify the practices to accommodate your particular needs.

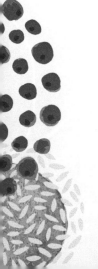

Yoga for a Sprained Ankle

TOTAL TIME: 10 MINUTES

GOOD FOR

This sequence focuses on using the arches of your feet to strengthen the muscles around your ankles.

REMEMBER Usually, an ankle is sprained laterally (on the outside) from rolling outwardly on the ankle. Through this series, focus on hugging your outer shins and ankles inwardly to engage the muscles that support the outside of the leg.

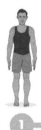

1

TADASANA
(see page 38): Hold for five centering breaths. Then, lift one foot off the floor at a time and hold for two more breaths.

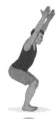

2

UTKATASANA
(see page 71): Exhale to sit into chair, then inhale to stand Tadasana. Repeat five times.

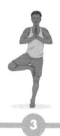

3

VRKSASANA
(see page 89): Hold for five breaths on each side.

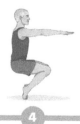

4

UTKATASANA WITH HEEL LIFT
(see page 82): Inhale, lift heels, exhale into "Toe Chair." Inhale, straighten legs: five times.

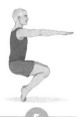

5

UTKATASANA WITH HEEL LIFT
(see page 82): Hold for 10 breaths.

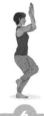

6

GARUDASANA
(see page 90): Hold for five breaths on each side.

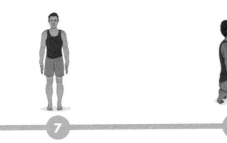

TADASANA
five centering breaths.

Optional: **VAJRASANA** (see page 88): If your injury is not new, you may elect to gently mobilize the ankle in a non-weighted position.

Yoga for a Rotator Cuff Injury

TOTAL TIME: 20 MINUTES

GOOD FOR

The rotator cuff is the capsule of muscles that hold the humerus bone in the shoulder socket. When recovering from a chronic injury, gentle movements in this joint can be helpful for maintaining mobility and encouraging blood flow.

REMEMBER During this practice, do not let your pain levels increase. Move your shoulder in an appropriate range of motion that gently invites mobility.

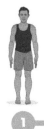

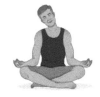

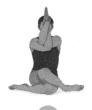

1

TADASANA
(see page 38): five centering breaths. Five shoulder rolls forward; five back.

2

SIMPLE NECK STRETCHES
(see page 30):
five breaths for each stretch.

3

GARUDASANA ARMS
(see page 32):
five breaths on each side.

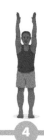

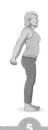

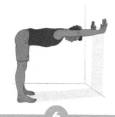

4

URDHVA HASTASANA
(see page 34): Inhale to reach arms forward and up, exhale to lower. Repeat five times.

5

YOGA MUDRA
(see page 33):
Hold for five breaths with each interlock.

6

SPINAL STRETCH AT THE WALL
(see page 40):
10 breaths.

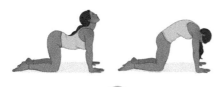 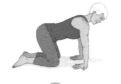 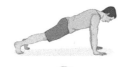

CAT/COW POSE
(if weight bearing is appropriate) (see page 50): 10 rounds. Inhale for Cow, exhale for Cat.

WRIST STRETCH
(see page 60): five breaths.

PHALAKASANA
(if weight bearing is appropriate) (see page 58): five breaths.

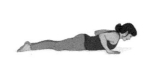 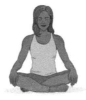

BHUJANGASANA
(see page 42): Hold for one breath. Repeat five times.

SUKHASANA
(see page 78): five centering breaths.

Yoga for a Torn Hamstring

TOTAL TIME: 25 MINUTES

GOOD FOR

This sequence works the hamstrings and the backs of the legs, helping bring blood flow and strength back to the injured tissue.

REMEMBER This sequence deliberately includes long holds to build strength in your glutes and hamstrings. Focus on keeping the weight in your heels and actively pulling your heels toward you in poses like Virabhadrasana Two, Parsvakonasana, and Setu Bandha Sarvangasana.

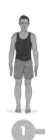 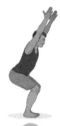 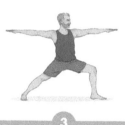

1

TADASANA
(see page 38):
five centering breaths.

2

UTKATASANA
(see page 71):
Hold for five slow
breaths. Repeat twice.

3

VIRABHADRASANA TWO
(see page 67): Hold
for 10 breaths on each
side. Repeat twice.

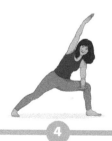 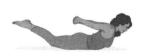 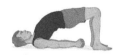

4

PARSVAKONASANA
(see page 68): Hold
for 10 breaths on each
side. Repeat twice.

5

SALABHASANA
(see page 44):
Hold for three breaths.
Repeat five times.

6

**SETU BANDHA
SARVANGASANA**
(see page 51): Hold for five
breaths. Repeat twice.

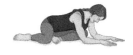 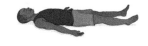

EKA PADA KAPOTASANA
(see page 75) or
THREAD THE NEEDLE
(see page 76): Hold for 10
breaths on each side.

SAVASANA
(see page 39):
five minutes.

Yoga for an Injured Achilles Tendon

TOTAL TIME: 15 MINUTES

GOOD FOR

This sequence strengthens and stretches the calves and may be appropriate once you have recovered from an acute state of an injury.

REMEMBER This sequence deliberately includes long holds to build strength in your glutes and hamstrings. Focus on keeping the weight in your heels and actively pulling your heels in toward you.

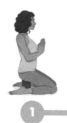 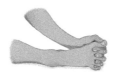 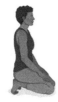

1

2

3

VIRASANA
(see page 83):
five centering breaths.

YOGI TOE MASSAGE
(see page 92): one
minute per foot.

VAJRASANA
(see page 88): Hold for 10 seconds, then release and tap out
the tops of feet. Repeat once.

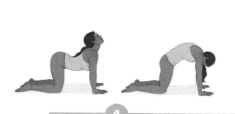 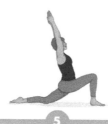 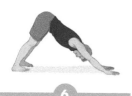

4

5

6

CAT/COW POSE
(see page 50):
10 rounds. Inhale for
Cow, exhale for Cat.

LOW LUNGE
(see page 70): Hold for five
breaths on each side, back
toes tucked or untucked.

ADHO MUKHA SVANASANA
(see page 65): Hold for 10
breaths, gently pedaling the
feet to stretch the calves.

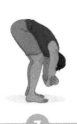 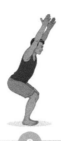 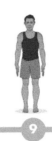

7

UTTANASANA
(see page 64):
10 breaths.

8

UTKATASANA
(see page 71):
five breaths.

9

TADASANA
(see page 38): inhale to
straighten your legs into
Tadasana, exhale to sit into
chair. Repeat five times.

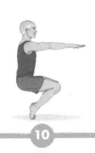 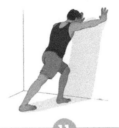 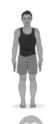

10

**UTKATASANA
WITH HEEL LIFT**
(see page 82): Inhale to lift
your heels, exhale to sit
into "Toe Chair." Inhale to
straighten your legs, exhale to
lower your heels and stand in
Tadasana. Repeat five times.

11

**MODIFIED
VIRABHADRASANA ONE**
(see page 84):
Hold for five breaths
on each side.

12

TADASANA
five centering breaths.

Yoga for Wrist Arthritis or Carpal Tunnel Syndrome

TOTAL TIME: 10 MINUTES

GOOD FOR

This sequence mobilizes and adds gentle weight to the hands and wrists. With chronic arthritis, careful mobilization can often help the joints, but be cautious that your pain levels do not increase. If putting weight on your wrists and hands is too uncomfortable, try the sequence for Hands-Free Yoga (see page 156).

REMEMBER This sequence deliberately puts weight on your hands and mobilizes your joints. When putting weight on your hands, press into your index finger mound and fingertips to distribute pressure evenly through your whole hand. If you have carpal tunnel syndrome, focus on pressing more weight into the base on your knuckles and fingertips to take weight out of the heel of your hand (you can also practice on your fingertips or fists).

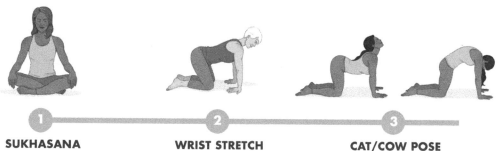

1

SUKHASANA
(see page 78): five centering breaths. Repeat, gently rolling your wrists and opening and closing your fists.

2

WRIST STRETCH
(see page 60): one hand at a time or both hands.

3

CAT/COW POSE
(see page 50): 10 rounds. Inhale for Cow, exhale for Cat.

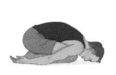

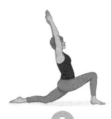

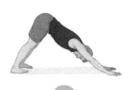

BALASANA WITH ARMS REACHING FORWARD
(see page 41): five breaths.

LOW LUNGE
(see page 70):
five breaths on each side.

ADHO MUKHA SVANASANA
(see page 65): 10 breaths
(can substitute Cat/
Cow Pose if you wish).

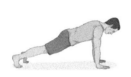

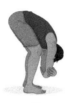

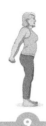

PHALAKASANA
(see page 58): two breaths,
then rest in Virasana (see
page 83). Repeat twice.

UTTANASANA
(see page 64):
10 breaths.

TADASANA
(see page 38) with Yoga
Mudra (see page 33): five
breaths with each interlock.

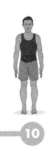

TADASANA
five centering breaths.

Hands-Free Yoga

TOTAL TIME: 40 MINUTES

GOOD FOR

This sequence is completely non–weight bearing on the hands and is perfect for anyone recovering from hand, wrist, or shoulder injuries.

REMEMBER This sequence puts weight on your hands and wrists. Make sure to take a wide stance in your standing poses (Virabhadrasana Two and Parsvakonasana) to reap the leg-strengthening benefits. Feel free to practice near a wall for support.

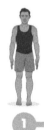
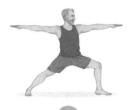
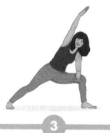

1

TADASANA
(see page 38):
five centering breaths.

2

VIRABHADRASANA TWO
(see page 67):
five breaths on each
side. Repeat once.

3

PARSVAKONASANA
(see page 68):
five breaths on each
side. Repeat once.

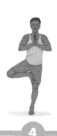
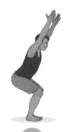
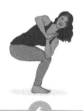

4

VRKSASANA
(see page 89):
five breaths on each side.

5

UTKATASANA
(see page 71):
five to 10 breaths.

6

PARIVRTTA UTKATASANA
(see page 55):
five breaths on each
side. Inhale to lengthen
and exhale to twist.

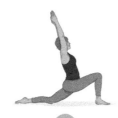

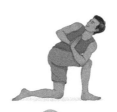

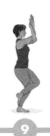

(7)

HIGH OR LOW LUNGE
(see page 70):
five breaths on each side.

(8)

**PARIVRTTA
PARSVAKONASANA**
(see page 54): five breaths
on each side. Inhale to
lengthen and exhale to twist.

(9)

GARUDASANA
(see page 90):
five breaths on each
side. Repeat once.

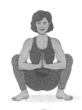

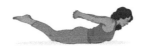

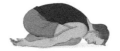

(10)

MALASANA
(see page 85):
10 breaths.

(11)

SALABHASANA
(see page 44):
five breaths. Repeat twice.

(12)

BALASANA
(see page 41):
10 slow breaths.

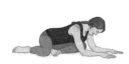

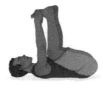

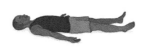

(13)

EKA PADA KAPOTASANA
(see page 75) or Thread
the Needle (see page 76):
10 breaths on each side.

(14)

ANANDA BALASANA
(see page 77):
10 breaths.

(15)

SAVASANA
(see page 39):
five minutes.

Chair Yoga

TOTAL TIME: 40 MINUTES

GOOD FOR

This sequence is designed to be done with a chair and wall for additional support. It is perfect for those with mobility and balance concerns.

REMEMBER Rather than "resting" in the chair, use it as a support for finding greater stability, length, and space in your body.

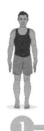

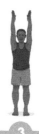

1

TADASANA
(see page 38):
five centering breaths.

2

SIMPLE NECK STRETCHES
(see page 30):
five breaths for each stretch.

3

**URDHVA HASTASANA
(WITH SIDE STRETCH)**
(see page 34): Hold each
side for five breaths.

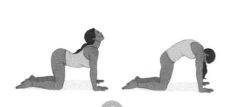

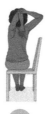

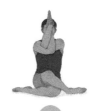

4

CAT/COW POSE
(see page 50):
10 rounds. Inhale for
Cow, exhale for Cat.

5

GOMUKHASANA ARMS
(see page 31):
five breaths for each side.

6

GARUDASANA ARMS
(see page 32):
five breaths for each side.

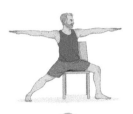

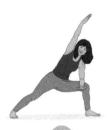

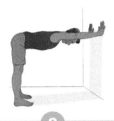

7

VIRABHADRASANA TWO
(see page 67):
10 breaths for each side.

8

PARSVAKONASANA
(see page 68):
five breaths for each side.

9

**SPINAL STRETCH
AT THE WALL**
(see page 40):
10 breaths.

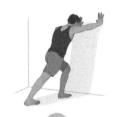

10

**MODIFIED
VIRABHADRASANA
ONE (WALL)**
(see page 84):
10 breaths for each side.

11

**PARIVRTTA UTKATASANA
(SITTING IN CHAIR)**
(see page 55):
five breaths for each side.

12

USTRASANA
(see page 48):
three breaths.
Repeat twice.

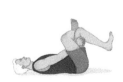

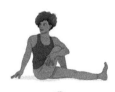

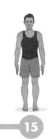

13

**THREAD THE
NEEDLE (CHAIR)**
(see page 76): five
breaths on each side.

14

ARDHA MATSYENDRASANA
(see page 52): five breaths
on each side. Inhale to
lengthen, exhale to twist.

15

TADASANA
five centering breaths.

Yoga for Spinal Issues

TOTAL TIME: 20 MINUTES

GOOD FOR

This sequence focuses on keeping the spine long and neutral to create traction and space without stressing the intervertebral discs.

REMEMBER In this sequence, focus on keeping the spine neutral (neither folding forward nor bending back), and use the strength of your legs for support. When you lie in Supta Hasta Padangusthasana, keep the entire back and back of your pelvis evenly anchored into the floor.

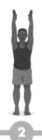

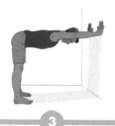

1

TADASANA
(see page 38):
five centering breaths.

2

URDHVA HASTASANA
(see page 34):
five breaths.

3

**SPINAL STRETCH
AT THE WALL**
(see page 40): 10 breaths.
Repeat twice.

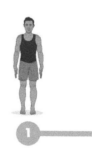

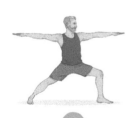

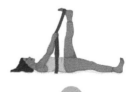

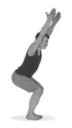

4

UTKATASANA
(see page 71):
10 breaths.

5

**VIRABHADRASANA
TWO**
(see page 67):
five breaths on each
side. Repeat once.

6

**SUPTA HASTA
PADANGUSTHASANA**
(see page 73):
five breaths for
each leg stretch.

7

SAVASANA
(see page 39):
five minutes.

Yoga for Disc Issues

TOTAL TIME: 20 MINUTES

GOOD FOR

If you have been diagnosed with a posteriorly bulging or herniated disc, your doctor may suggest core engagement and gentle backbends to support the imbalance. Not all disc issues are the same; please check with your doctor first before using this sequence to ensure that it's right for you.

REMEMBER In Plank Pose, ensure that your low back is not dropping to the floor; use your core strength to lift the front of your body toward the back of your body. When you lie in Supta Hasta Padangusthasana, keep your entire back and the back of your pelvis evenly anchored into the floor.

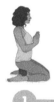
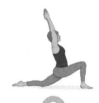
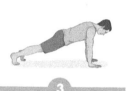

VIRASANA
(see page 83):
five centering breaths.

LOW LUNGE
(see page 70):
five breaths on each side.

PHALAKASANA
(see page 58):
five to 10 breaths.

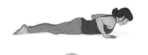
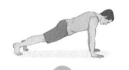
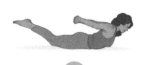

BHUJANGASANA
(see page 42):
three breaths. Repeat
five times.

PHALAKASANA
five to 10 breaths.

SALABHASANA
(see page 44):
three breaths. Repeat
three times.

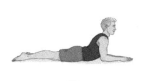 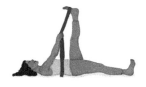 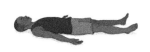

7

SPHINX POSE
(see page 46):
10 breaths.

8

**SUPTA HASTA
PADANGUSTHASANA**
(see page 73): 10 breaths
for each leg stretch.

9

SAVASANA
(see page 39):
five minutes.

Yoga for a Knee Replacement

TOTAL TIME: 25 MINUTES

GOOD FOR

This sequence is designed for those who have had a knee replacement and have been approved for activity. The sequence includes mobility and strengthening exercises for the knee to support your recovery.

REMEMBER Work mindfully to keep weight even in the four corners of your feet and your knees aligned with your ankles (particularly in Parsvakonasana, High Lunge, and Setu Bandha Sarvangasana). Move slowly to stabilize and strengthen the muscles around the knee.

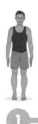
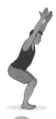
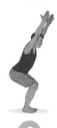

1
TADASANA
(see page 38):
five centering breaths.

2
UTKATASANA (ACTIVE)
(see page 71): Exhale to sit into chair, inhale to stand in Tadasana (see page 38). Repeat 10 times.

3
UTKATASANA
(passive): five breaths.

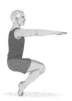
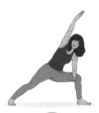
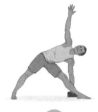

4
UTKATASANA WITH HEEL LIFT
(see page 82):
five breaths. Repeat once.

5
PARSVAKONASANA
(see page 68):
five breaths on each side. Repeat once.

6
TRIKONASANA
(see page 69):
five breaths on each side.

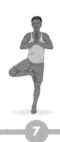

7

VRKSASANA
(see page 89):
five breaths on each side.

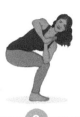

8

PARIVRTTA UTKATASANA
(see page 55):
five breaths on each
side. Inhale to lengthen
and exhale to twist.

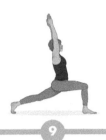

9

HIGH LUNGE
(see page 70):
10 breaths on each side.

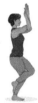

10

GARUDASANA
(see page 90):
five breaths on each side.

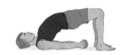

11

**SETU BANDHA
SARVANGASANA**
(see page 51):
five breaths. Repeat twice.

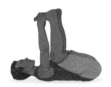

12

ANANDA BALASANA
(see page 77):
10 breaths.

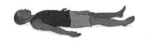

13

SAVASANA
(see page 39):
five minutes.

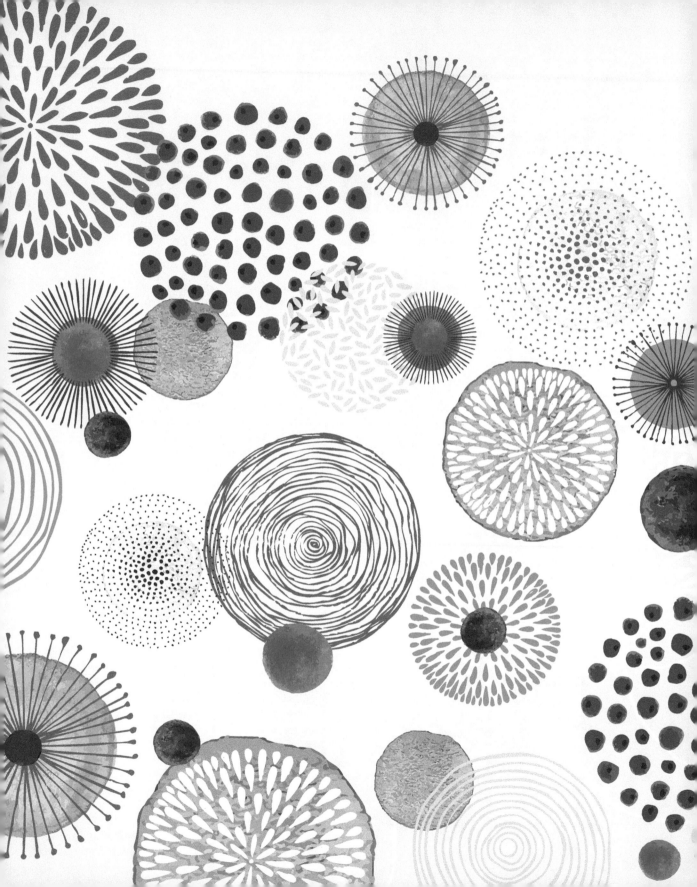

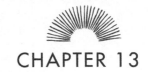

Aches and Pains

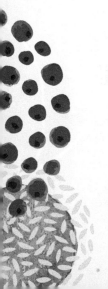

Yoga for Headaches

TOTAL TIME: 15 MINUTES

GOOD FOR

This sequence stretches the neck and shoulder muscles that may encourage tension headaches when they get tight.

REMEMBER Keep your chest open, shoulders relaxed away from your ears, and the back of your neck long.

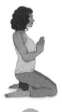

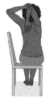

① VIRASANA
(see page 83), Sukhasana (see page 78), or seated in a chair: five centering breaths.

② SIMPLE NECK STRETCHES
(see page 30): five breaths for each stretch.

③ GOMUKHASANA ARMS
(see page 31): five breaths on each side.

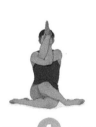
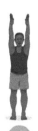
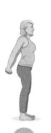
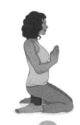

④ GARUDASANA ARMS
(see page 32): five breaths on each side.

⑤ URDHVA HASTASANA
(see page 34): five breaths.

⑥ YOGA MUDRA (SEATED)
(see page 33) or Tadasana (see page 38): five breaths with each interlock.

⑦ VIRASANA, SUKHASANA, OR SEATED IN A CHAIR:
five centering breaths.

Yoga for a Stiff Neck

TOTAL TIME: 15 MINUTES

GOOD FOR

Neck tightness often originates from the chest and shoulders. This sequence stretches the chest and shoulder muscles that may encourage a stiff neck.

REMEMBER When practicing backbends, draw your upper arms back to widen your collarbones and release the muscles at the back of your neck.

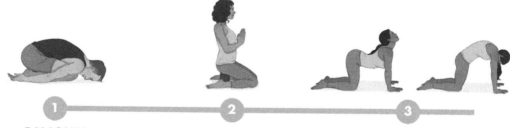

BALASANA
(see page 41):
five centering breaths.

VIRASANA
(see page 83) with Simple
Neck Stretches (see page 30):
five breaths for each stretch.

CAT/COW POSE
(see page 50):
10 rounds. Inhale for
Cow, exhale for Cat.

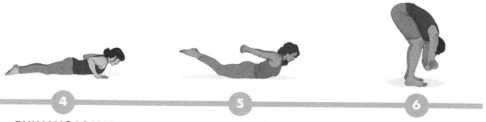

BHUJANGASANA
(see page 42):
five breaths. Repeat twice.

SALABHASANA
(see page 44): five breaths
(optional: have hands in
Yoga Mudra; repeat twice).

UTTANASANA
(see page 64):
10 breaths. Release the
weight of your head.

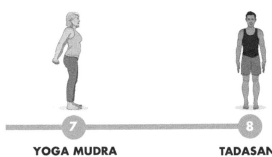

YOGA MUDRA
(see page 33): five breaths.

TADASANA
(see page 38): five centering breaths.

Yoga for Tight Shoulders

TOTAL TIME: 20 MINUTES

GOOD FOR

This sequence moves the shoulder joint in all directions to fully mobilize the joint and relieve tightness.

REMEMBER During this sequence, focus on the movement of your arm bone (humerus) in your shoulder socket, and keep your neck and facial muscles relaxed.

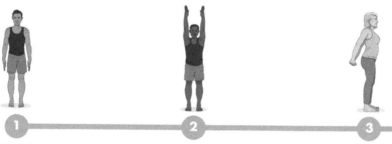

TADASANA
(see page 38):
five centering breaths.

URDHVA HASTASANA
(see page 34):
five breaths.

YOGA MUDRA
(see page 33):
five breaths.

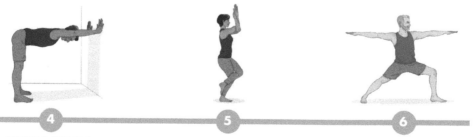

**SPINAL STRETCH
AT THE WALL**
(see page 40): 10 breaths.

GARUDASANA
(see page 90):
five breaths on each side.

VIRABHADRASANA TWO
(see page 67):
five breaths on each side.

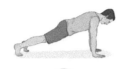

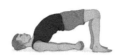

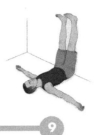

7

8

9

PHALAKASANA
(see page 58):
five breaths.

**SETU BANDHA
SARVANGASANA**
(see page 51): five
breaths. Repeat once.

VIPARITA KARANI
(see page 93):
five minutes.

Yoga for a Tight Upper Back

TOTAL TIME: 25 MINUTES

GOOD FOR

The upper back often feels tight, weak, and sore from bad postural habits. This sequence strengthens the upper back muscles that support upright posture and healthy alignment.

> **REMEMBER** During this backbending sequence, focus on how your shoulder blades and upper back are feeling. As you move into each backbend, remember to draw your shoulder blades together and spread your chest.

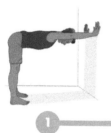

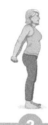

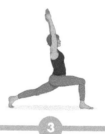

**SPINAL STRETCH
AT THE WALL**
(see page 40):
10 centering breaths.

YOGA MUDRA
(see page 33):
five breaths with
each interlock.

HIGH LUNGE
(see page 70):
10 breaths on each side.

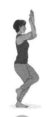

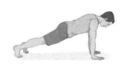

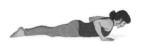

GARUDASANA
(see page 90):
five breaths on each side.

PHALAKASANA
(see page 58):
five to 10 breaths.

BHUJANGASANA
(see page 42):
five breaths. Repeat twice.

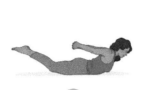

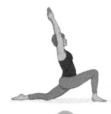

SALABHASANA
(see page 44):
five breaths. Repeat twice.

LOW LUNGE
(see page 70):
five breaths on each side.

USTRASANA
(see page 48):
three breaths. Repeat once.

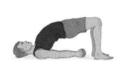

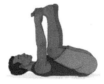

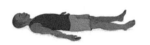

**SETU BANDHA
SARVANGASANA**
(see page 51): five
breaths. Repeat twice.

ANANDA BALASANA
(see page 77):
10 breaths.

SAVASANA
(see page 39):
five minutes.

Yoga for a Sore Low Back

TOTAL TIME: 20 MINUTES

GOOD FOR

The low back can become compromised by poor posture and pelvic position. This sequence helps both stretch the hamstrings and strengthen your postural muscles to support a healthy low back.

REMEMBER When in a forward folding pose (Uttanasana and Prasarita Padottanasana), bend your knees to hinge from your hips rather than allowing your spine to overly arch.

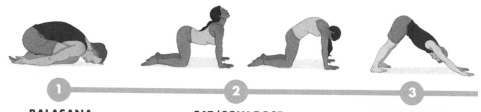

BALASANA
(see page 41):
five centering breaths.

CAT/COW POSE
(see page 50):
10 rounds. Inhale for
Cow, exhale for Cat.

**ADHO MUKHA
SVANASANA**
(see page 65): 10 breaths
(you can substitute Cat/
Cow Pose if you wish).

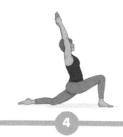

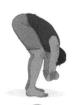

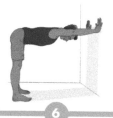

LOW LUNGE
(see page 70):
five breaths on each side.

UTTANASANA
(see page 64):
10 breaths.

**SPINAL STRETCH
AT THE WALL**
(see page 40):
10 breaths.

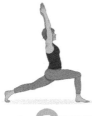

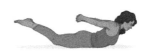

7

HIGH LUNGE
(see page 70):
five breaths on each side.

8

PRASARITA PADOTTANASANA
(see page 72):
10 breaths.

9

SALABHASANA
(see page 44):
five breaths. Repeat twice.

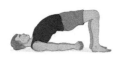

10

SETU BANDHA SARVANGASANA
(see page 51): five
breaths. Repeat twice.

11

ANANDA BALASANA
(see page 77):
10 breaths.

12

SAVASANA
(see page 39):
five minutes.

Yoga for Tight Hips

TOTAL TIME: 30 MINUTES

GOOD FOR

This delicious sequence focuses on opening the muscles surrounding the hips.

REMEMBER During this sequence, focus on how your thigh (femur) is moving in its socket, and explore taking it through its full range of motion.

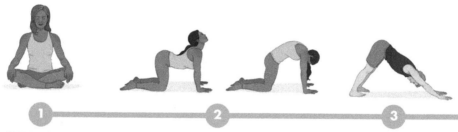

SUKHASANA
(see page 78): Hold for five breaths. Add Uttanasana (see page 64); take five breaths. Recross legs, repeat.

CAT/COW POSE
(see page 50):
10 rounds. Inhale for Cow, exhale for Cat.

ADHO MUKHA SVANASANA
(see page 65): 10 breaths (you can substitute Cat/Cow Pose if you wish).

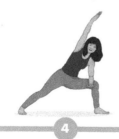
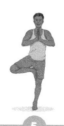
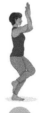

PARSVAKONASANA
(see page 68):
10 breaths on each side.

VRKSASANA
(see page 89):
five breaths on each side.

GARUDASANA
(see page 90):
five breaths on each side.

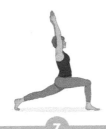
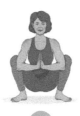
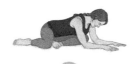

HIGH LUNGE
(see page 70):
five breaths on each
side. Repeat once.

MALASANA
(see page 85):
10 breaths.

**EKA PADA
RAJAKAPOTASANA**
(see page 75) or Thread
the Needle (see page 76):
10 breaths on each side.

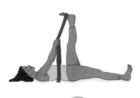
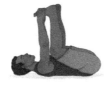
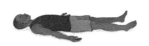

**SUPTA HASTA
PADANGUSTHASANA**
(see page 73): Hold each
stretch for five to 10 breaths.

ANANDA BALASANA
(see page 77):
10 breaths.

SAVASANA
(see page 39):
five minutes.

Yoga for Sore Legs

TOTAL TIME: 30 MINUTES

GOOD FOR

This sequence targets the muscles of the feet, calves, and thighs to relieve muscle tension and soreness.

REMEMBER Be mindful when stretching your feet and calves. Find a place where you can still soften into—rather than resist—the stretch.

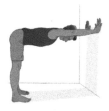

1

VIRASANA
(see page 83):
five centering breaths.

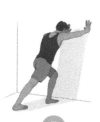

2

VAJRASANA
(see page 88): five breaths,
then tap out the top of
your feet. Repeat once.

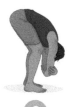

3

UTTANASANA
(see page 64):
10 breaths.

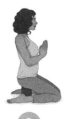

4

**SPINAL STRETCH
AT THE WALL**
(see page 40):
10 breaths.

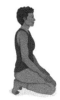

5

**MODIFIED
VIRABHADRASANA ONE**
(see page 84):
five breaths on each side.

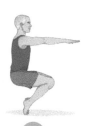

6

**UTKATASANA
WITH HEEL LIFT**
(see page 82):
five breaths. Repeat twice.

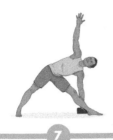
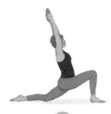
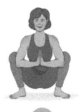

7

TRIKONASANA
(see page 69):
five breaths on each side.

8

LOW LUNGE
(see page 70):
five breaths on each
side. Repeat once.

9

MALASANA
(see page 85):
10 breaths.

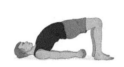
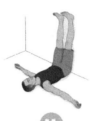

10

**SETU BANDHA
SARVANGASANA**
(see page 51):
five breaths. Repeat twice.

11

VIPARITA KARANI
(see page 93):
five minutes.

Yoga for Sore Hands

TOTAL TIME: 15 MINUTES

GOOD FOR

This sequence is designed to gently mobilize and strengthen your hands and wrists.

REMEMBER This sequence has several poses that require putting weight on your hands. Make sure to press down through the tips of your fingers and anchor your index finger firmly down to evenly distribute the weight through the whole hand.

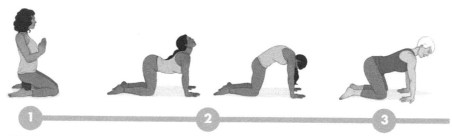

VIRASANA
(see page 83) or
Sukhasana (see page 78):
five centering breaths.

CAT/COW POSE
(see page 50):
10 rounds. Inhale for
Cow, exhale for Cat.

WRIST STRETCH
(see page 60):
five breaths. Repeat twice.

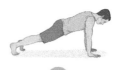
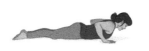
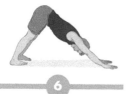

PHALAKASANA
(see page 58):
five to 10 breaths.

BHUJANGASANA
(see page 42):
five breaths. Repeat twice.

**ADHO MUKHA
SVANASANA**
(see page 65): 10 breaths
(you can substitute Cat/
Cow Pose if you wish).

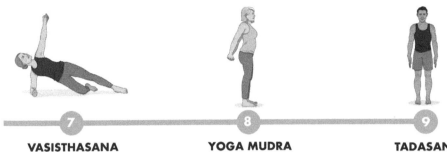

VASISTHASANA
(see page 59):
five to 10 breaths on each side.

YOGA MUDRA
(see page 33): five breaths
with each interlock of hands.

TADASANA
(see page 38): five
centering breaths.

Yoga for Poor Posture

TOTAL TIME: 40 MINUTES

GOOD FOR

Poor posture is often caused by a weak core and tight hamstrings. This sequence targets opening the hamstrings while strengthening the back and abdominal muscles to improve posture and functional alignment.

REMEMBER When practicing backbends, engage your core (abdominals) by knitting your lower belly toward your spine to support the low back.

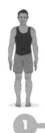 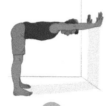 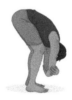

1   **2**   **3**

| **TADASANA**
(see page 38):
five centering breaths. | **SPINAL STRETCH
AT THE WALL**
(see page 40): 10 breaths. | **UTTANASANA**
(see page 64):
10 breaths. |

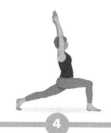 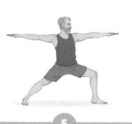 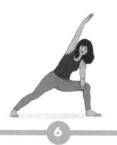

4   **5**   **6**

| **HIGH LUNGE**
(see page 70) with Yoga
Mudra (see page 33): five
breaths for each side. | **VIRABHADRASANA TWO**
(see page 67):
five breaths on each
side. Repeat once. | **PARSVAKONASANA**
(see page 68):
five breaths on each
side. Repeat once. |

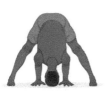

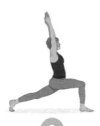

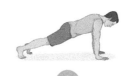

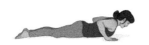

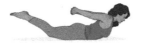

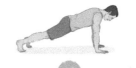

7

8

9

**PRASARITA
PADOTTANASANA**
(see page 72):
10 breaths.

HIGH LUNGE
five breaths on each
side. Repeat once.

PHALAKASANA
(see page 58):
five to 10 breaths.

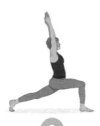

10

11

12

BHUJANGASANA
(see page 42):
five breaths. Repeat once.

SALABHASANA
(see page 44):
five breaths. Repeat once.

PHALAKASANA
five to 10 breaths.

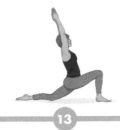

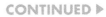

13

14

CONTINUED ▶

LOW LUNGE
(see page 70)
with Yoga Mudra:
five breaths on each side.

USTRASANA
(see page 48):
three breaths.
Repeat twice.

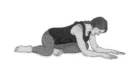

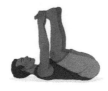

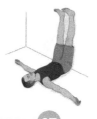

15

EKA PADA KAPOTASANA
(see page 75) or Thread
the Needle (see page 76):
10 breaths on each side.

16

ANANDA BALASANA
(see page 77):
10 breaths.

17

VIPARITA KARANI
(see page 93):
10 breaths.

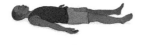

18

SAVASANA
(see page 39):
five minutes.

Yoga for General Flexibility

TOTAL TIME: 40 MINUTES

GOOD FOR

This well-rounded sequence is designed to provide a gentle, whole-body opening.

REMEMBER In each posture, focus on creating more space by reaching from the center of your body out through your extremities. Use your breath to create more space in your body.

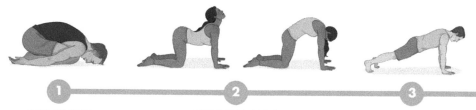

BALASANA
(see page 41):
10 centering breaths.

CAT/COW POSE
(see page 50):
10 rounds. Inhale for
Cow, exhale for Cat.

PHALAKASANA
(see page 58):
five to 10 breaths.

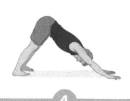
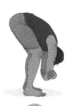
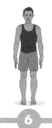

**ADHO MUKHA
SVANASANA**
(see page 65): five to 10
breaths (you can substitute
Cat/Cow Pose if you wish).

UTTANASANA
(see page 64):
10 breaths.

TADASANA
(see page 38):
five breaths.

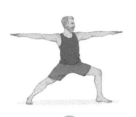

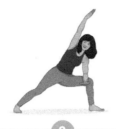

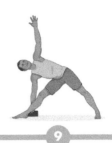

7

VIRABHADRASANA TWO
(see page 67):
five breaths on each
side. Repeat once.

8

PARSVAKONASANA
(see page 68):
five breaths on each
side. Repeat once.

9

TRIKONASANA
(see page 69): five breaths
on each side. Repeat once.

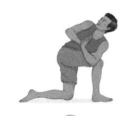

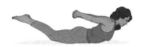

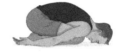

10

**PARIVRTTA
PARSVAKONASANA**
(see page 54): five breaths
on each side. Repeat once.

11

SALABHASANA
(see page 44):
five breaths. Repeat twice.

12

BALASANA
10 breaths.

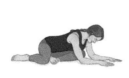

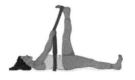

13

**EKA PADA
KAPOTASANA**
(see page 75, or
76): 10 breaths
on each side.

14

ANANDA BALASANA
(see page 77):
10 breaths.

15

**SUPTA HASTA
PADANGUST-
HASANA**
(see page 73): Hold
each stretch for five
to 10 breaths.

16

SAVASANA
(see page 39):
five minutes.

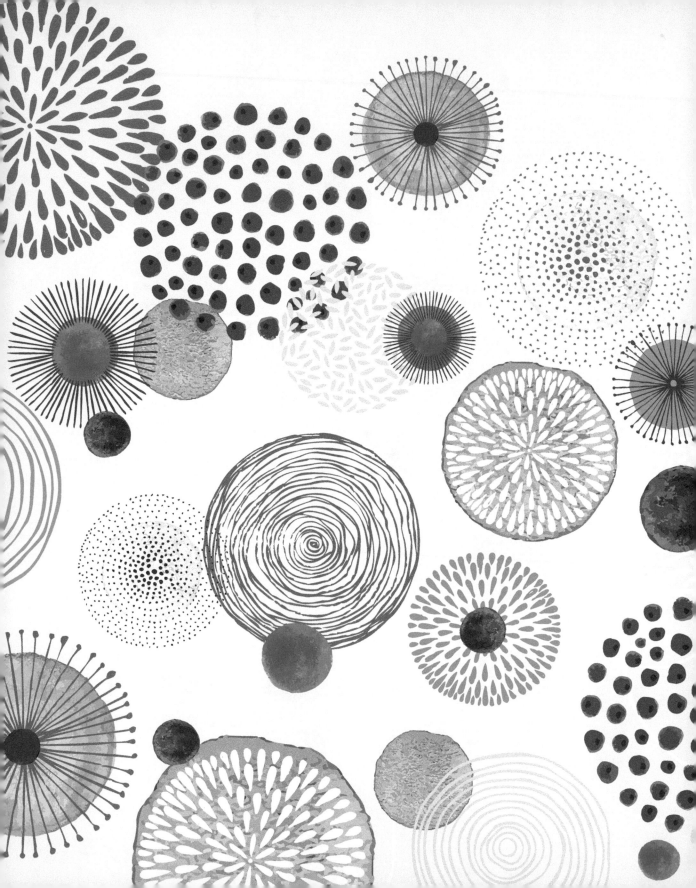

CHAPTER 14

Customize Your Yoga Practice

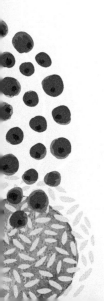

Once you have a grasp of the postures and the sequences, you can begin to create your own! Become your own teacher and feel free to design new sequences and variations for your own body's needs. There is no right way to do yoga; the most important aspect of the practice is cultivating your own mindfulness and committing to your own self-care.

TIPS FOR SEQUENCING

As you begin to create your own sequences, here are some tips to keep in mind:

START WITH A GROUNDING POSE. Begin every sequence with a stable seated, standing, or reclined pose (Tadasana [see page 38], Savasana [see page 39], Sukhasana [see page 78], Virasana [see page 83], or Balasana [see page 41]). Take a few deep breaths before you start to check in with your body, breath, and emotions.

WARM UP. As you start your practice, incorporate a few poses that build heat, such as standing poses (Low Lunge and High Lunge [see page 70], Virabhadrasana Two [see page 67], or Utkatasana [see page 71]), to warm up your big muscles.

ADD ONE OR TWO BALANCING POSES. Balance is an important component of physical health. Incorporate at least one balancing pose into your sequence to build your ankle strength.

DO EASIER POSES FIRST. As you build a sequence, do the more accessible poses first to warm your body up before increasing the complexity.

INCORPORATE AT LEAST ONE BACKBEND. Daily life tends to have us living in "slumpasana!" By incorporating at least one backbend (Bhujangasana [see page 42], Ustrasana [see page 48], or Salabhasana [see page 44]), you will ensure that you are activating and strengthening your back muscles, which help keep your spine tall and strong.

STRETCH AND RELAX. At the end of every sequence, enjoy a couple of stretching poses like Thread the Needle (see page 76) or Ananda Balasana (see page 77).

ALWAYS DO SAVASANA. If you're doing a longer sequence, always end with a centering pose and a few more mindful breaths or, better yet, rest in Savasana (see page 39) for at least five minutes.

SEQUENCING INSPIRATION

When creating your new sequences, the sky is the limit! Here are some tips for keeping it fresh.

+ Target a certain part of your body. Create a sequence that uses poses primarily from a chapter in part 2 to really focus on that area.

+ Cultivate a well-rounded sequence. Create a sequence by choosing two poses from each chapter in part 2 to make sure you're hitting all the different areas of your body.

+ Change the rhythm. A quick sequence will feel very different than a slow sequence. Return to your favorite sequences and change the pace of your movements. Take note of what you find.

+ Listen to what your body needs. Choose poses that directly target the areas of your body that require the most attention.

+ Write down all the names of the poses. This will make it easy to pick and choose the poses you want to include on a given day.

+ Practice your least-favorite poses. We tend to focus on poses that we really enjoy, but often the poses that we dislike are actually the ones that we need.

+ Share with friends. Create a yoga group where you can practice with friends. You can each create new sequences to share.

+ Check out free online classes to get inspired. You can come practice with me at doyogawithme.com and get some new ideas!

Resources

WEB

Here are some great online resources for your continuing practice:

✦ Visit my website (rachelyoga.com) or my YouTube channel (youtube.com/rachelscottyoga) for tips.

✦ Practice with me for free online at Do Yoga With Me (doyogawithme.com) and get more sequencing ideas.

✦ *Yoga Journal:* yogajournal.com.

✦ Silver Sneakers: classes for older adults on YouTube; search for "Silver Sneakers" on YouTube.

BOOKS

Here are a few of my favorite yoga philosophy books that you may enjoy:

✦ *The Heart of Yoga: Developing a Personal Practice* by T. K. V. Desikachar

✦ *Light on Life: The Yoga Journey to Wholeness, Inner Peace, and Ultimate Freedom* by B. K. S. Iyengar

Here are a few books on yoga poses that you may also enjoy:

✦ *30 Essential Yoga Poses: For Beginning Students and Their Teachers* by Judith Hanson Lasater

✦ *The Breathing Book: Good Health and Vitality Through Essential Breath Work* by Donna Farhi

✦ *Relax and Renew: Restful Yoga for Stressful Times* by Judith Hanson Lasater

✦ *Wit and Wisdom from the Yoga Mat: 125 Peaceful Poses, Mindful Musings, and Simple Tricks for Leading a Zen Life* by Rachel Scott

References

Cartee, G. D., et al. "Exercise Promotes Healthy Aging of Skeletal Muscle." *Cell Metabolism* 23, no. 6 (June 2016), 1034–47. http://doi.org/10.1016/j.cmet.2016.05.007.

Hood, D. A., et al. "Maintenance of Skeletal Muscle Mitochondria in Health, Exercise, and Aging." *Annual Review of Physiology* 81, no. 1 (February 2019), 19–41. http://doi.org/10.1146/annurev-physiol-020518-114310.

Niedziałek, I., et al. "Effect of Yoga Training on the Tinnitus Induced Distress." *Complementary Therapies in Clinical Practice* 36 (August 2019), 7–11. http://doi.org/https://doi.org/10.1016/j.ctcp.2019.04.003.

Ponte, S. B., et al. "Yoga in Primary Health Care: A Quasi-Experimental Study to Access the Effects on Quality of Life and Psychological Distress." *Complementary Therapies in Clinical Practice* 34 (February 2019), 1–7. http://doi.org/10.1016/j.ctcp.2018.10.012.

Seo, D. Y., et al. "Age-Related Changes in Skeletal Muscle Mitochondria: The Role of Exercise." *Integrative Medicine Research 5*, no. 3 (September 2016), 182–6. http://doi.org/10.1016/j.imr.2016.07.003.

Sherrington, C., et al. "Exercise for Preventing Falls in Older People Living in the Community." *Cochrane Database of Systematic Reviews* 1 (January 2019). http://doi.org/10.1002/14651858.CD012424.pub2.

Index

About the Author

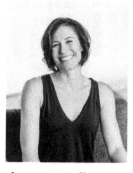 Rachel Scott is a yoga educator, author, and instructional designer. She helps yoga teachers and studios thrive in their businesses and share their passion for yoga with their students. In addition to her published books, Scott has contributed to *Yoga International*, *Huffington Post*, and numerous podcasts. She has also presented at yoga conferences all over North America.

As a teacher, she loves helping her students create strong, balanced, smart yoga practices that make them feel healthy and vibrant in all areas of their lives. A lover of philosophy, she continually wrestles with the juicy bits of life—relationships, love, and personal development—and blogs regularly about how yoga can support our lives off the mat. You can connect with her on social media @rachelscottyoga, visit her on her website at rachelyoga.com, or practice with her online at doyogawithme.com. She is also a wicked coffee drinker and lover of all furry creatures.

CPSIA information can be obtained
at www.ICGtesting.com
Printed in the USA
LVHW021452070220
646024LV00003BC/3